COME LIVE WITH ME

BARBARA K. KINCAID

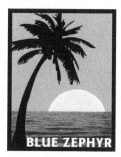

San Francisco

COME LIVE WITH ME

A Memoir of Family, Alzheimer's, and Hope

DEDICATION

In Grateful Memory of
Ann Loeb Bronfman

CONTENTS

PREFACE

Why I Write: For Alzheimer's Family Caregivers

In 2000, my mother Dixie Garrett Kincaid was diagnosed with probable Alzheimer's. I should not have been surprised. My grandmother had it, as did my mother's older sister. Though I hoped our family might be spared, eventually I became my mother's sole caregiver.

I read the statistics on caregiving stress and its impact on the health of family caregivers. In 1999 the Journal of the American Medical Association (JAMA) published a landmark study, "Caregiving as a Risk Factor in Mortality..." The study documented that caregivers who experienced caregiver strain had mortality risks that were sixty-three percent higher than the non-caregiver control group. Mortality risks remained for four years.[1]

That was other people—not me, I thought. I was healthy and careful to get check-ups on time. I was wrong. Alzheimer's is a family disease. Not contagious, but it might as well be since over time it has the power to generate other illnesses through burnout and stress. So to people who think Alzheimer's is just an old person's disease and, let's face it, not worthy of too much time, attention, or public investment: think again.

More recent research suggests there may be benefits from family caregiving. Generally, the advantages come from the focus and stimulation required in managing care for another. However, the complexity and diversity of caregiving tasks make it hard to quantify in a research setting. The newer data, reported by Paula Span in an article in *The New York Times in 2011*, modified the impact of family caregiving.[2] Epidemiologist Lisa Fredman of Boston University reported

---

1. Richard Schulz and Scott R. Beach, "Caregiving as a Risk Factor for Mortality: The Caregiver Health Effects Study," *Journal of the American Medical Association 282*(23) (1999): 2215-2219.

2. Paula Span, "Caregiving's Hidden Benefits," *The New Old Age* (blog), *The New York Times*, October 12, 2011, http://newoldage.blogs.nytimes.com/2011/10/12/caregivings-hidden-benefits/

that the physical and mental activities required by caregiving could be beneficial to family caregivers. Dr. Fredman acknowledged that the results of her study were skewed somewhat by the fact that caregivers were self-selected.

Each Alzheimer's experience is different. If there is one lesson that I would shout from the rafters, it is this: *If you've seen one case of Alzheimer's—you've seen one case.* That was and is the mantra of a terrific support group that I discovered in 2004, and that wisdom has come home time after time.

Alzheimer's is terminal. There is no cure, no guaranteed way to prevent it. Roughly five million have the disease in the US. About fifteen million are family caregivers,[3] ranging from daily hands-on care to visiting family members in assisted living facilities. More than seventy percent of unpaid family caregivers are women. Each circumstance has its own stress: money management, caregiving training and competency, the emotional intelligence or lack of it in health care providers, and those who interact with the patient and the caregiver. It is often a story of careers ended sooner than anticipated to assume the role of caregiver 24/7.

Medications helped manage the disease. I was grateful to have prescriptions for my mother that were not available for my grandmother and my mother's older sister. They made a difference for my mother, but they don't for everyone. Even for us, the impact was limited.

My mother required twenty-four-hour care for ten years, but she undoubtedly had the disease for an additional ten to twelve, with milder symptoms. Care in Alzheimer's units of assisted living easily runs from $40,000 to $100,000 a year (in 2010 dollars), depending on the region of the country and the level of care. Even in my version of "sweat equity care", there were expenses in excess of $20,000 a year for day care, transportation, supplies, and occasional nursing assistants.

Forecasters paint a bleak picture for the future. As boomers age and the number of eighty-five-year olds increases, the number with

3. Alzheimer's Association, "2011 Alzheimer's Disease Facts and Figures," http://www.alz.org/downloads/facts_figures_2011.pdf.

Alzheimer's is expected to climb to at least seven million by mid-century.[4] So, I write to share my experience with the hope of giving some comfort to those who choose to be a caregiver. Eyes-wide-open empowerment. I also write for therapy, and to expose some of the boneheaded behaviors that I have witnessed in the "helping professions." You can't make this stuff up.

It is ironic that the basis for this Alzheimer's story is memory and memoir. The genre is an odd choice for stories about Alzheimer's, which steals reason along with the good and bad memories of one's life experience—a necessary basis for human connection. It must be acknowledged, of course, that memoir is often based only on the writer's point of view and is therefore highly subjective. In some cases, I have changed the names of people and organizations, particularly when I have been highly subjective, critical, and without mercy. *Yes, this is a confession.* In other cases, individuals have died and I did not feel comfortable using names without their permission. Much of the time names stayed in the book, if for no other reason than a very public acknowledgement to those who contributed so much to my peace of mind.

Family caregiving is tough, physically demanding work. I won't kid you. But it is also rewarding. There are untold moments of joy and laughter that deserve to be shared. Late at night, for example, I carved out some personal time for myself. I discovered a wholeness to my single life as I cared for Mother and Dad. Sometimes my life choices seemed fine, logical, and acceptable; sometimes they seemed poor, counter-productive to the point of being self-destructive. Finding wholeness and forgiveness—especially self-forgiveness—was totally unanticipated. Caregiving must be an exercise in self-examination. What do I do well? What do I do poorly? Honestly. Candidly. My journey will not be your journey. Nonetheless, I am firmly committed to sharing what I learned about caregiving and, in the process, about myself.

I hope you will smile, maybe even laugh... feel some sadness here and there, but above all believe in your own ability to find a path that will work for you and your loved one. Laugh. Cry. Believe. That's it—the human experience.

---

4. "Alzheimer's Data," (presented at 2nd Alzheimer's Association International Conference on Prevention of Dementia in Washington, DC, June 10, 2007).

DIRGE WITHOUT MUSIC[5]

EDNA ST. VINCENT MILLAY

I am not resigned to the shutting away of loving hearts in the hard ground.
So it is, and so it will be, for so it has been, time out of mind:
Into the darkness they go, the wise and the lovely. Crowned
With lilies and with laurel they go; but I am not resigned.

Lovers and thinkers, into the earth with you.
Be one with the dull, the indiscriminate dust.
A fragment of what you felt, of what you knew,
A formula, a phrase remains,—but the best is lost.

The answers quick and keen, the honest look, the laughter, the love,
They are gone. They have gone to feed the roses. Elegant and curled
Is the blossom. Fragrant is the blossom. I know. But I do not approve.
More precious was the light in your eyes than all the roses in the world.

Down, down, down into the darkness of the grave
Gently they go, the beautiful, the tender, the kind;
Quietly they go, the intelligent, the witty, the brave.
I know. But I do not approve. And I am not resigned.

AUTHOR'S NOTE: A high school English teacher used the last line to describe me. I hated it, of course, but I lived my life proving her right. "I know. But I do not approve. And I am not resigned."

---

5. Edna St. Vincent Millay, "Dirge Without Music" in *Collected Poems*, edited by Norma Millay (Harper & Row, 1956). Reprinted with permission of The Permissions Company, Inc., on behalf of Holly Peppe, Literary Executor, The Millay Society. www.millay.org.

COOKIES IN HER PANTS

It's a good thing my mother, Miss Dixie, is dead. Otherwise some of the things I report here would kill her.

She was adamant. She and my father Hiram were not going to the long-term care community in the town next door. Try as I might to sell it, Mother wasn't buying. If they went there, she said, "He'll go talk to people and just leave me (in the apartment)." In fact, her point was hard to argue with. I could see that their residency might work that way.

At the time, I was visiting from Virginia. We were sitting at the dining room table in Michigan, talking, and out of my mouth it came.

"Why don't you come live with me?" *What in blazes did I just say?*

"Okay," she replied. *Now you've done it. There's no turning back.*

That's how it happened. I just sort of blurted it out and it was done. I had not been consciously considering it as an option. But once I said it, bringing them into my house felt like the right thing to do. That's how I became an Alzheimer's 24/7 family caregiver, two years after my mother's diagnosis and as my father's health began to fail. On a cold November evening in St. Louis, Michigan, my life changed as I blurted out that proposal.

*

My mother's given name was Dixie. As Alzheimer's slipped in, she became Miss Dixie. A social worker created her handle at her Arlington County day care program. It was a perfect fit. Her Alzheimer's persona contained traces of the original woman, but now she was generally more likable, humorous, and charming. Yes, MORE likeable. When she was contented or engaged, her eyes were bright and shining.

One Sunday afternoon, I heard the shuffle of feet and saw a sweet little white-haired, five-foot woman headed toward me in the kitchen. "Where's my horse?" she asked.

Think fast, I said to myself. "Where did you last see it?"

"Well, I don't know." And off we went into la-la land.

Black-haired and vivacious as a young woman, Miss Dixie now had snow-white hair in her Alzheimer's days. She still had great skin and a beautiful smile throughout, not to mention a wit. Before Alzheimer's, my mother could be sad and depressed. With the illness, she was cheerful and played jokes. As she was helped down the stairs, she would pretend to jump. Then, she'd turn to her helper with a smile and twinkle in her eye, happy with her tease and her helper's reaction to it.

Before Alzheimer's, my mother could be demanding and opinionated. When I was in college, my mother called my newspaper boss to tell him he was working me too hard. Appalled by her intervention, I was grateful not to be fired. With Alzheimer's, Miss Dixie was not judgmental and forgot how to manipulate. She couldn't remember how to play those games. Unlike the old days, her feelings weren't hurt if people didn't agree with her. She just forgot about it.

So many of the things that she craved as Dixie, she no longer cared about with Alzheimer's. She might have liked the idea of a designer bag as a younger woman. But when I just eliminated her handbag as something else to lose—she never noticed.

Life was simpler. She loved food, including healthy vegetables and fruits, music, being with other people, and rides in the country. As we headed out the door, she would turn to me. "Why don't you drive?" She was oblivious to the fact that she had not had a driver's license in a very long time.

But then, I would pull into a parking spot in front of a specialty store and she would perk right up. "Ice cream," she said correctly, with shining eyes and a happy smile.

Forgetfulness was a *great* relief on many issues. She no longer followed "Judge Judy" or required members of the household to listen to the judge. In the late stages of Alzheimer's she didn't like noise, but she would watch football on television, noting what "a good job those boys did keeping their uniforms clean." Despite not quite getting the game, she was contented watching football and golf on television, a habit she had cultivated for more than sixty-five years with my father. And she won prizes for playing golf and bingo at day care.

There were old movies, too. She liked musicals with Judy Garland, Fred Astair, and Gene Kelly. When I wondered sometime whether she was enjoying a particular film, I would see her foot moving to the music, confirming her pleasure.

On television, she liked Emeril Lagasse on the Food Network. She could recognize food and still loved vibrant colors. Plus, she liked his personality and the music on his old shows. I once made the mistake of asking her a question while Emeril was on and got a quick "shush."

Miss Dixie could not remember that she had lived in Michigan for fifty-nine years. But, she knew she had grown up in West Virginia.

"I want to take this to Mother," she told me after lunch one Sunday afternoon as she folded a brightly colored piece of paper. "Okay," I said. What was the point of making her sad by reminding her that her mother had been dead thirty years?

After my dad died and she began to forget his death, she asked: "Where's Hiram?"

"West Virginia," I said, failing to note that the true location was Clover Cemetery.

"Oh," she said. She moved away from the conversation easily.

There was sweetness, but there was also a sort of reckless self-preservation that would have appalled Dixie. The judgmental Dixie would have let her Alzheimer's self know about her disapproval. When words became hard for her to find—she kicked. She hit and even bit. That behavior would have shocked the Dixie who was my mother. Still, she met Alzheimer's on her own terms. No sad crying for her; more likely a right hook every now and then.

One of my favorite pictures was at the age of five, barefoot, smiling and holding her doll. Also in the picture was her brother Richard, who was roughly a year and a half younger. Wearing a sailor suit, no doubt made by hand by Grandmother, he stood *very* straight and looked *very* serious—already playing the part of quality Air Force material.

Even as a ninety-year-old with advancing Alzheimer's, that little girl was with us. As I carefully guided Miss Dixie into bed, she liked to bounce up and down on the mattress, swing her legs, and smile.

As her language skills disappeared, she developed new communication tools. When she was happy, she would smile and clap her hands and pat someone sweetly when she was being guided down the hall. No words necessary. Similarly, she communicated her displeasure when she didn't want to get out of bed by pushing one's hand away.

"Mine" would sometimes be her only verbal expression as Alzheimer's progressed. It was most often said in anger with a jerk or a light slap. It might be a tissue, an extra carton of milk, or, heaven forbid, a cookie. In the early stages, she could be a cookie pusher. A guest for tea would be offered the plate of sweets over and over.

Winter or summer, Miss Dixie always had a hat on. Her gloves, a winter mainstay, might stay on even while she ate crackers at day care.

"She didn't like us much today," the activities director explained as Miss Dixie sat away from the group with her hat, coat, gloves, and a doll baby over her shoulder, all while she munched snack crackers in her own little world.

Both Dixie and Miss Dixie loved color. As she grew older—red, hot pink, purple, and black became her favorites. She was right; she looked best in those colors. I dressed her in "mom" jeans and long-sleeved polo shirts for "school," Mother's name for adult day care.

I often found surprises when I got her ready for bed. One night while my dad was still alive I found a cookie wrapped in plastic in her underpants. *You just never knew when you're going to need a cookie!*

And that became our new family joke. Out for a car ride with Mother and Dad, looking for a restaurant, "Sure wish I had a cookie in my pants," my dad said.

*

With Alzheimer's I could count on her loving bright green steamed broccoli and carrots for supper. The colors made her happy; so happy, in fact, that she sometimes demanded I take a picture of her dinner plate before she ate. In traffic she might say, "That's a pretty car." Red, in all its various shades, was her favorite.

Most of the time, but certainly not all of the time, Miss Dixie was cheerful and accepting of Alzheimer's. She expected to have it, because her mother had it. "It could be worse," she told me soon after she was diagnosed. She had made her peace early on with her disease and her fate, while I had not.

Dixie and Miss Dixie kept intact a sense of showmanship. Zipping hurriedly out of a grocery store and heading toward Mother in the car in the handicapped spot, I came to look forward to her royal wave. "I'm here," was the message of her perfectly executed signal. It was also one of the things I missed most after she was gone. That and our dinners together, but I'm getting ahead of my story.

I'M AN ONLY

I'm five years old tomorrow. It's also VJ Day. Last year Daddy took a picture of me with my doll's bed on the porch, holding my doll and my fingers in a V. I had my pajamas on so it must have been early, and the sun was in my eyes.

My friend Bethie lives downstairs. I'm not happy right now. I had the sweetest teddy bear. He was brown with black button eyes and a red yarn mouth. Bethie killed him. She threw him down the stairs and his head came off. Mother sewed his head back on, but it's not the same. So, I'm staying away from Bethie. I loved my bear. I had him for a long time and took really good care of him, too. Mother said I did and that she guessed that might be because I was an only child. Bethie has an older sister, Margaret. Mother says Margaret is a brat. That's where Bethie learns bad things, Mother says. Killing Teddy was mean and I'm disappointed in Bethie. I don't think I'm going to ask her to come for birthday cake or my tea party with the dolls tomorrow.

We live across from the park. I used to live in West Virginia, but now I live in Michigan. The town is St. Louis and I think the area is called central Michigan. We have windows that go almost to the floor so I can stand in the window and see kids playing on the teeter totters and swings. I can even see the park when I play in our rocking chair, rocking back and forth really fast. Actually, I don't do that so much anymore since I fell out of the chair last year and cut my eyebrow. I have a scar over the left one. I was going fast in the chair. Then, the next thing I knew I was on the floor with a gash over my eye. I got scolded. The blood made Mother upset. I was a little scared, but now I've settled down quite a bit.

Our floors are hardwood and shiny; Mother keeps them that way. That means they are slick, too. Great for scooting in your sock feet. The *windows have white curtains with ruffles that Mother irons sometimes. They're quite pretty.*

In the winter, a woman who looks like a ladybug walks on the park sidewalk. Her coat is brown with black dots on it. Her hair is white. I showed the ladybug to Mother and she laughed. Said she was a high school teacher, not a ladybug. English teacher, she thought. Her name was Miss Deline.

Mother is homesick: she tells me that often. It seems to make her sad. Unlike me, she has five brothers and two sisters. She writes to Grandmother a lot and Grandmother writes back. That helps Mother keep up with what's going on, but I'm not sure it helps her not be sad. I wish I could help.

*

Hmm, memories. I've been channeling my earlier self tonight. Late at night is my time for reflection. For as long as I can remember I hated being an only child. I played by myself, talked to myself, and then I learned to read. I was still alone, but I wasn't as lonely. I could escape to other lands and places, quickly. By the time I discovered the public library in grade school, Mother and Dad both worked in their dry cleaners and we lived out of town, not in a neighborhood with sidewalks and foot traffic. So, I learned to entertain myself very early; newspapers, books, and magazines. In the summertime, I'd check out several books at a time from the library. I even enjoyed reading the *World Book Encyclopedia* that the folks bought for my homework desk to help with schoolwork. I used to read the encyclopedia and our *Webster's* dictionary for fun, believe it or not. No wonder my test scores were pretty good.

My bitterness about being an only child would only emerge when outsiders made assumptions. They assumed that only children had cushy lives. That we were waited on hand and foot. That whatever we wanted, we got. I found that offensive. I had chores. I vacuumed, dusted, and cooked meals. Not very well, mind you. But, I had stuff to do full time from the age of twelve. I'm quite certain my responsibilities started before that, given there was some kind of learning curve. But I don't remember precisely when. My chores also included lunch in the summer time and mowing a very large lawn that took almost two hours with a power mower. Whenever someone spoke about how spoiled only children were, I nearly blew a gasket. Only when I got to college and discovered there were kids who actually didn't know how to do laundry did I lay off the chore thing. It was one of my only-child talking points, which had more to do with assumptions and biases than the actual chores.

Then, there was my rebellious phase, which was most of junior high and high school. Now that I think about it, it was probably sixth grade, too. My dad told me my mind and attitude "went to hell when we got television." We waited a long time before getting one. I can remember the whole family, all three of us, going to friends' houses on Saturday night to watch television shows like *Your Hit Parade* with the Lucky Strike extras. Then, we got our very own set.

I loved it. Like all the housewives twice my age, junky soap operas were my thing. Plus *American Bandstand* in the late afternoon. Normally I was supposed to be vacuuming. (We lived in the basement of a house that was going to be built.) *Click. Oops, that's the upstairs door. Here comes Dad. Hurry, hurry.* Dad would roar in from the dry cleaning shop next door and see the vacuum cleaner sitting in middle of the floor. He'd yell. Scream. And probably swear. Disconnect the TV antenna and leave. I'd hustle over to the television and hook the antenna back up. *In business again.* I was fast. I would hear him coming in the door upstairs. Boom. The set was off. While my peers were allegedly into sex, drugs, and rock 'n roll, I was taking the TV apart. *Dull, boring.*

During those rebellious times, I craved a sibling to blame for the unwashed dishes and the floor that wasn't vacuumed and the TV that was on. *Poor me.* Then, there was life I envisioned for myself. I wanted a career, but I also wanted a houseful of kids.

Christmas holidays were always a little sad. Mother and Dad were terrific, don't get me wrong, but I craved that Hallmark picture with lots of people showing up around the table. I even wrote a story about being a career woman and later marrying a man with children. That was the way I saw my life emerging; that was my fix for being "an only."

My blame game continued during the seven years it took me to get an undergraduate degree. I wanted a large school as an escape from small town life. I loved the anonymity. Yet, so much of the time I felt overwhelmed and in over my head. I had good grades in high school and miserable grades in college. I assumed I was supposed to get mediocre marks because I came from a small town. Besides, I had to work so I *couldn't* do well academically. *Oh, please. How tedious and uninteresting that whine is.* (This was one of my victimization phases.) Very late in my college career I started knocking off top grades with four-point terms. But I had already blown my chances for graduate school with miserable grades earlier. I was mildly content with a D in some economics class. Re-take the course and get a better grade? *Are you nuts?* Graduate school was the last thing on my mind. All I wanted was to get the hell out of school with a bachelor's degree. My expectations for myself were low and my confidence was compromised. After all, I was a member of the Silent Generation. I lacked the bravado of the Boomers. So, as an only child, shouldn't all of this have been easy for me? I thought life was cushy for only children?

Then, there were my downward spirals. My biggest one happened when I lived in Philadelphia. Before my dad gave up big city driving, he and Mother made the trip at Christmas time. He arrived with a painful lump on his knee. They didn't have a family doctor then, so I scheduled an appointment with mine. A cyst was drained and he went on bed rest with heat and anti-inflammatory medications. Clearly, age was becoming an issue and neither parent seemed to know when to go to the doctor. It bothered me and tapped into my melancholy tendencies and childhood fears about being an only and/or becoming an orphan. After each visit, I had a weepy meltdown hidden from everyone's view except my own. Would this be the last time I saw one or both? Anticipatory grief. *Shrink time again!*

ECCENTRICITIES OR ALZHEIMER'S?

"I'm getting Alzheimer's," my mother would tell me on the phone in the early 1990s. I was living in Philadelphia. "What makes you think that?" I would ask. My question was dumb for anyone who was beginning to lose processing skills. She couldn't explain. Then, I would tell her she didn't have Alzheimer's. The truth, of course, was that I was in denial. Despite discounting my mother's observation, I remembered my grandmother's history of Alzheimer's and I was careful to explore the information readily available about the disease. This was before a robust Internet, so information was more limited. Occasionally there were Alzheimer's reports in the media. As a recovering news junkie, I picked up those reports. I used the information to reassure myself that Mother didn't have Alzheimer's. The truth was, I wasn't ready for her to have Alzheimer's. I had career obligations.

As certain as I felt that my mother did NOT have Alzheimer's, she was becoming more difficult and odd in some ways. It was not memory particularly, or at least I couldn't pinpoint it as memory. It was more flawed reasoning and thinking. First, she had a very bad fall tripping over a vacuum cleaner. I arranged for her to visit me in Philadelphia for medical tests, but there was no diagnosis other than severe disc disease in her spine. I was certain her additional complaints of fatigue and mobility discomfort were real. As a younger adult, Dixie had had terrible headaches—headaches that I now believe were probably undiagnosed migraines. The medical school where I worked as a fundraiser was doing continuing education and grand rounds sessions on fibromyalgia. Much of what Mother described fit those symptoms, but we never got it pinned down. Her complaints gradually subsided, possibly when Alzheimer's started to take over.

Before Alzheimer's kicked in, Mother was a miserable sleeper. She would sleep a few hours in her lounge chair. When Dad got some extra money, he bought an adjustable bed, which permitted her to crawl into a bed that was configured much like the lounge chair. She began sleeping much better. Dad was understandably proud that his investment made a difference.

Mother also began to get more difficult and strange in conversations, which were mostly limited to the telephone. Dad and she might visit twice a year, once in the summer and once at Christmas time. As a fundraiser, the end of the tax year sometimes required my presence in the office. So as an accommodation to my schedule, they did the holiday traveling.

After one trip to Philadelphia, my dad told me the travel was getting too hard on him and I needed to think about coming to Michigan instead. My mother dismissed the idea that driving was difficult for my dad. This was a typical pre-Alzheimer's response. Judgmental. "Oh, we can still make the trip." Did she help drive? No. But she knew better than he or me or anyone. I also suspected the house was in such disarray that she didn't want me to see it. When I was a kid, she blamed the messiness on me. Sometimes appropriately. Sometimes not so much. Either way, her scapegoat was out of the house now.

My dad was also growing increasingly exasperated with her difficulty in getting ready for a trip. Packing requires memory and skill in sequencing. Even as a young woman, my mother was habitually late. So, it was difficult to see her behavior as a characteristic of Alzheimer's. When I was in my early twenties and lived near East Lansing in Okemos, Michigan, my mother arrived at my apartment for Sunday dinner four hours late. No apology. No explanation. She was sure it wouldn't matter. WRONG! That was the self-absorbed and self-centered Dixie. Not all the time, but enough of the time to be memorable. Her indifference to her own behavior and its impact on other people enraged me as a kid when I felt particularly powerless.

Anyway, once she came to visit in Philadelphia she wrapped every piece of my jewelry that she could find in plastic wrap, while I was at work. You could probably hear me scream up and down the Mainline. Dixie remained certain that encasing my jewelry in sticky see-through stuff was a good idea. No wonder she was always late. Taking sticky stuff off your jewelry when you're trying to get to the office in the morning would make me late, too. I should have seen this as an example of impaired judgment and an early symptom of Alzheimer's, but I didn't know enough about the early symptoms.

"Hi, what are you doing?" her cheery voice on the phone asked one day. "Well, Mother, I'm packing for that business trip I told you about," I said.

"Oh, where are you going again?"

"California. Los Angeles and San Francisco."

"Hmm, what are you going to do?" she said.

I would explain. We would chat about the weather, or occasionally current events, or sports, since she followed sports with my dad. She liked basketball player Charles Barkley, who got himself into hot water from time to time.

"Charles didn't really mean that," she would explain. "He was just messing around."

"Tell me again where you're going?" she asked. I repeated. "How long will you be gone?" I repeated.

Inevitably the conversation would take place after ten o'clock and there would be at least three repeats of my travel plans. Still, I didn't get it. I was focused on MY work. Was she trying to drive me nuts? That was my explanation. It didn't occur to me, perhaps because I didn't want to consider it, that the conversation might be fueled by the beginning of Alzheimer's. The repetitions were memory related, but I wasn't ready to see that.

One evening her telephone call mentioned a "slight" auto accident she'd had. Her description focused on the driver of the other car leaving the body shop driving the "wrong" way. *What?* I asked myself. *Never mind, I have work to do.*

"I think he has Alzheimer's," she announced, referring to the other driver. "Oh," said I moving on. Then, all of a sudden, Dixie no longer wanted to drive. My dad always speculated that she might have gotten lost coming back from a shopping trip twenty miles away. So, one potentially unpleasant situation—taking the keys and telling the patient that he or she should no longer drive—was avoided. Still, I didn't connect this new circumstance with Alzheimer's. It could just have been an age-related preference.

Later, we had a completely nonsensical telephone conversation about people stopping by the house to talk to Dad. It made no sense at all, but I was in a hurry and needed to do something, so I put the incident out of my mind. In fact, the conversation was a confabulation, a mixture of reality and imagination, and a term I would later learn as part of my Alzheimer's vocabulary.

Even though Dad was reluctant to take on big city driving, he still was comfortable heading to West Virginia for reunions with his siblings. Indeed, he needed to renew that connection regularly and Mother enjoyed it, too. I would drive over from the Northern Virginia area to Spencer, the county seat of Roane County, about fifty miles from Charleston. We'd meet up at the reunion/family gathering at Dad's oldest brother's home on Memorial Day.

One of Mother's memory aid techniques was a little red notebook with all of the family names, especially the children. She refused to join the group without her notebook for quick reference before she said hello to folks face to face. That alone should have been a signal for me, but it wasn't.

On one visit I was lolling in the kitchen over coffee when I learned that my Dad, frustrated with her pace of getting ready, had left my mother in Michigan. Just flat out left her. I remembered calling the house and mentioning that I thought she was in West Virginia.

"No, I'm here," she said, matter-of-fact. No mention that Dad was in West Virginia. Nothing. Sitting in the kitchen in Spencer was the first I'd heard about this trip with my aunt and uncle laughing. *Hmm*, I thought.

The next day, as Mother was getting ready to leave, I went to the apartment where they stayed. My dad was elsewhere. I listened and watched. It *was* her memory; she couldn't remember from one minute to the next where she was in packing and getting herself ready. Sequencing was an enormous challenge for Alzheimer's patients, but I didn't know that yet. Nonetheless, the light was beginning to dawn on me. *I'm not ready for this*, I heard my inner voice say.

Months passed. It was February 2000. Dad's oldest living brother died after years of illness. I knew my father would be racked by the loss. The brothers shared the same birthday; Dad was seven years younger. Hobe had a dry cleaning business, and Dad modeled his business after Hobe's. Dad would laugh later in life as he noted that Hobe's financial success didn't come from the cleaners, but his investments in oil and gas.

"I forgot to notice that until it was too late," he would say as he shrugged his shoulders and smiled.

I drove to West Virginia for the funeral services.

When I arrived at the house, my mother was there with a neighbor trying to figure out how to work the coffee maker. I didn't think too much about that, but then she introduced me as living in Tennessee. *What the...? Tennessee. Never even been there. Let alone live there. Talk about la-la land.* It was smack in front of me now. I couldn't ignore it or pretend that it wasn't happening. *The problem was memory, dementia, Alzheimer's.*

FROM WEST VIRGINIA TO MICHIGAN

Dixie Gail Garrett met Lester Hiram Kincaid in high school in the 1930s, maybe on the school bus ride to Spencer. Her ride was eighteen miles and his, ten. Both were country kids who were smart and from large families. His siblings numbered twelve, with ten children who lived, and Dixie had had five brothers and two sisters. All of the Garrett babies were hardy and lived. So did their parents, until ages eighty-eight and ninety.

After high school in West Virginia, my mother went to business school. Like Mother, Dad, who used his middle name, was attractive. Together they were a memorable couple. In one of my favorite photos, Dad looked like a 1950s movie star. A natural athlete, he attended Morris Harvey College in Charleston on a football scholarship. He quit school and went to work a semester before he graduated, a decision he regretted all his life. His mother, his last surviving parent, had just died when he made the decision, a bad one as he saw it years down the line. In my tumultuous college years, his greatest worry was that I would do as he did: quit before I got a degree.

A year and a half after my paternal grandmother's death, my parents married in August 1939. I was born four years later. When I was three years old the family relocated to Michigan, where my dad worked for Michigan Chemical. How they made the decision to move remained a bit of a mystery to me. Finding a job in post-World War II was, to say the least, different. Word of mouth seemed an important recruitment tactic. The industrialized North was becoming a drawing card in areas of Appalachia, including West Virginia. Dad worked for a chemical plant in South Charleston, as did a handful of other Michigan transplants. Rumor had it there were good jobs in chemicals in Michigan. So, a few men took off on a train without their families to test the new environment. The gamble paid off. Later, their families supported one another through the transition, resulting in lifelong friendships. Michigan Chemical in those days was a thriving enterprise.

One of the odd contradictions about my dad was his strong anti-union stance. In the early years, he spoke of John L. Lewis with complete disdain. He used to say that the power of Lewis in West Virginia was the reason he left West Virginia. Maybe it was the wartime coal strike that Lewis led, but my dad despised labor unions. Yet, he moved to Michigan, where labor unions, particularly in the metropolitan areas, were influential and dominant. And he was a silent Democrat. Anti-union, but pro-working man or woman, my own family was an introduction to the curious inconsistencies that I discovered about US politics.

Small black and white photographs with my father's handwriting on the back described the best-looking houses in St. Louis. The advance man was clearly trying to "sell" my mother on the community. I don't think she ever really believed she had a choice. How hard it must have been for her to leave that boisterous, entertaining family of hers. I realize that I never understood the depth of her loss and homesickness. She said it often enough. Even though I was young, I remember her melancholy. Still, I couldn't really understand how uprooted and lost she felt.

The details of how we got from Michigan Chemical to the dry cleaning business are fuzzy, too. But it happened. Dad was "gassed" in some manufacturing mishap, and he decided to get out of the chemical business. Well, kind of. Based on the success of his older brother's dry cleaning business in West Virginia, Dad decided to try the chemicals of dry cleaning and take that business model to central Michigan.

Mother and Dad went into the business when I was about five. Both worked very hard and the work was extremely physical. My dad was very good with the chemicals and the big machines for cleaning and tumbling. He was also the guy who got the tough spots out. We lived next door to the cleaners, so I would get off the school bus, put my roller skates on, and skate through the two large rooms at the front of the dry cleaners. The back area with the large tumblers was off limits. The front of the building was my mother's domain. She was the alterations person, silk finisher, back-up press operator, and billing clerk.

Mother had learned to sew from Grandmother and an older sister, Lenore. Dixie was an extraordinary seamstress. Beginning as a teenager, she was recognized for her sewing first in home economics, then as people admired the clothes she made for herself and me. Her rules and processes were often extreme, or so it seemed to me. I watched her and asked why she was binding seams in a dress she was making for herself. The dress was lined and it was embroidered satin, an elegant, creamy beige with small coral flowers. She made a small coral silk hat to go with it. But why bind the seams? "Because that's the way to do it right," was her response. *Hmm,* I thought to myself, *sounds crazy to me. I want a dress to wear, not to look at the seams.* More all-nighters and the next thing I knew I had a nice dress, but my seams weren't bound and it wasn't satin, though as I grew older sometimes it was.

My mother had style and flair, too. One of my St. Louis friends, who later became a lifelong Washington, DC, friend—Tito Piccolo—used to call my mother Loretta Young after the movie and television actress. Beautiful with skill and charm—that was my mother.

In the beginning, my mother's brother Loman and his wife Madelyn were partners in the dry cleaning business. I don't remember how the partnership came about. Loman was recently returned from World War II (General George Patton's "Hell on Wheels") and probably open to new employment ideas. Dixie in her homesickness would have made a convincing case that Michigan could be fun and together they could make a go of it.

One of my early responsibilities was to ride in the delivery truck with Uncle Loman and tell him how to get to people's houses. I knew where folks lived since I had ridden with my dad. I had a good memory and sense of direction even though I was only five or six. There was only one seat for the driver in the truck so I would stand in the well of the door and play a human Global Positioning System (GPS).

"Barbara Kay," my uncle said. "There's a cat on that porch. Do you think that cat's gonna bite me?"

"No," I responded. "That's a nice cat."

"Okay," he said as he jumped from the truck. Sure enough, he came back alive. So my record as a cat psychologist was never challenged. Had I ever seen the cat before? Nah. I just felt certain at the age of six that the World War II hero would survive the porch kitty. The partnership in the dry cleaners lasted a couple of years. The war hero and his wife were homesick for West Virginia, too, and that became the downfall of the partnership.

MICHIGAN IN THE 1950S

Despite the hard work and long hours that my parents endured in those days, both parents were fun, good, and supportive in different ways. Road trips were always a big deal at our house. Beginning in the 1950s, Michigan had great roads in a large physically diverse state—the motor capital of the world.

It also had great lakes—the big ones, but what I remember most were the small ones. Fifteen miles from home where we could have a quick thrown-together picnic after a hot miserable day in the dry cleaning business. One of my favorite pictures of Mother and me was taken in Rock Lake. I was about five, had a life jacket on, and a whiny-looking face. My mother, who did not swim and was often very frightened of water, was smiling broadly and gamely trying to get her rotten little kid to cheer up. Not certain it worked on this occasion, but I certainly took swimming lessons later, including synchronized swimming or water ballet, which I hated.

Then, there were the big trips. "Up north," as we used to say. The UP, short for the Upper Peninsula. In the early 1950s there was only one way to get to the UP—by ferry. The Mackinaw Bridge didn't open until 1957. And the lines to get on the ferry on summer weekends were miles and miles. We got a place in line and stayed with the car. If we didn't, we'd have to start over for a wait that was often six hours in the summer. So, that was my first exposure to tailgating. The old picnic basket was heartily packed in the back of the station wagon. Mother's fried chicken, someone's potato salad or cole slaw. It was a homemade feast and yes, because it was such an ordeal to get across the bridge, there were often multiple families on the trip.

Then we got on this large wonderful ferry. We could feel the spray on our faces and watch the waves bounce us around. The UP was different from the lower peninsula. First, miles and miles of enormous trees. Towns were small and often were the result of settlements around mining areas in the earliest days.

Farm families would put out a sign welcoming travelers to stop and spend the night. "Tourist Rooms Vacancy" was what I looked for as the official spotter. Not nearly as swank as today's bed and breakfast places, but clean reasonably priced accommodations. Sometimes breakfast was included, sometimes it wasn't.

Every now and then, Dixie would play tour director in tourist homes. On one trip, two families were traveling in our car. The men slept apart from the women. Mother opened the door to the upstairs where the men slept and yelled, "Hit the deck. Rise and shine." Turned out there were lots of people up there, not just folks from our car, so we left much more quickly than anticipated to cover Mother's embarrassment, giggling softly on our hurried way out.

Dixie was also a stage mother. At six or seven, I was a tap dancer. I had forgotten all about my tap dancing career until I found a newspaper article when I was cleaning out my parents' house. Not quite the *Washington Post*, but the article in the *St. Louis* (Michigan) *Leader Press* explained that I provided entertainment at the Brownie Scout Christmas tea. I remembered my number: "Rudolph, the Red Nosed Reindeer."

Then there was my fabulous costume and the closing of my big number. Of course, Mother made my costume. She made almost everything I wore. Red satin pleated skirt. Square-necked white satin top. A big sparkling holiday bell that covered the entire front of my costume. I mean big, too. The fabric was finished with cheap glitter and the glitter always fell off. My big finish for Rudolph was a curtsy kind of bow right on "You'll go down in his-tor-y."

I used the same costume for Valentines' Day, but with a big sparkling heart in place of the bell. I think I danced to "Let Me Call You Sweetheart," although I don't remember whether I had a big finish.

The other thing you should know was that my mother, the stage mother in the making, used to carry a six-by-six-foot piece of linoleum in the back of the car so that I could perform at the drop of a hat. Her desire to be a stage mother, however, was disrupted significantly by my lack of talent. I only had two numbers that I remember. Or, it may be that I am already blessed with a flawed memory.

Holiday cookies were one of her amusing obsessions while I was in grade school. Recipe after recipe was tested for flavor that was just right. Cookie cutters were collected: many Santas (face and full suit), Christmas trees, Rudolph the Red-Nosed Reindeers, bells, tree ornaments and on and on.

There was a butter cookie base even for the cookies decorated with frosting. Dixie's treats needed to be works of art and have great flavor. There were also butter cookies that came from a cookie press and were sprinkled with colored sugars. Great brownie recipes, including a terrific butterscotch brownie, were part of her repertoire, too.

Christmas cookies had these additional attributes, according to Dixie. Even the Santas and Christmas trees should not be too large. They did not belong hanging on a tree, but on a sterling silver platter with a doily. Pressed cookies should be dainty in size. Large cookies were seen as graceless and inappropriate. Paper plates could be used for giving cookies away, but they should be wrapped in see-through with dramatic bows. I was the bow specialist, but truthfully they were ugly.

So many rules. As a result, I have never made a Christmas cookie in my life and never intend to. The cookie years were followed by the fruitcake years and the homemade mint years. All of these projects never really got under way until eleven o'clock at night and might end at four or five in the morning. These efforts were inevitably followed by complaints of exhaustion and the need for sympathy and compassion from her only child. Sometimes I measured up, sometimes not. If not, it was pointed out how ungrateful I was. After all, this was being done for ME. Didn't I need to take cookies to school? Yeah, but the paper didn't say butter cookies decorated as though they were being sold at Harrods Food Court in London. Well, things need to be done PROPERLY.

My dad was the go-to person on certain other matters. I was about eight and was being sexually harassed on the school bus. The terminology was different in those days. "Bothered" was probably the descriptor. A little creep named Marvin, who also happened to be the bus driver's son, was putting his arm around me and basically feeling me up. Marvin was at least two years younger than I was. He was short, dark haired, and had dorky thick glasses. I remember looking into the bus driver's mirror as he watched his rotten progeny do his thing. I was really angry that he let the little creep continue. But, behavior like that was tolerated in those days. It might have been dangerous to stop the bus at that point, but I also knew the jerk would do it again.

My cries of, "Leave me alone," weren't working. Forget my mother. She'd have some nicey-nice suggestion that would be totally ineffective with this guy. I needed a plan with an edge to it and Lester Hiram was the person to talk to.

So, leaving the bus I didn't even go through the front part of the dry cleaning plant where my mother was. I roared up the gravel driveway and headed to the back entrance, my dad's part of the shop. See, here's the thing about my dad: he wouldn't necessarily rule out a more aggressive physical approach. A former college football player with a hard-scrabble early life, he understood the rules for taking care of yourself. That I was a girl didn't matter. Or, indeed, it made it more imperative that I know how to handle myself, from his perspective.

Sure enough, my dad didn't disappoint. The next day I executed the plan.

Marvin made his move. I told him to stop. He didn't. I told him I would hit him with my lunchbox if he didn't. Regrettably he continued, so I let him have it. Crash! Bang! Glass shattered as I slammed my metal lunchbox over his head. Marvin got the message. I broke my thermos in the process. Quietly and quickly, Dad and I whipped out to buy a new thermos when I got home.

Not long after our thermos-buying spree, the bus driver showed up in the dry cleaners to report my slugfest.

"Yes," my dad said, "We've told her she has to warn the person before she retaliates and she said she did that." My mother was mortified. I hid and smiled secretly.

No further comment from the bus driver. Problem solved. Of course, were this to happen today, there would be court costs, lawyer fees, and so on.

Perhaps that was the beginning of my Scottish Warrior Princess persona, which came into play as I challenged folks who got in my way as I struggled to care for my mother and dad. Both of my parents could be fierce when crossed and I inherited a double dose of strong will, not to mention a work ethic.

The Diagnosis

After my mother introduced me as living in Tennessee, I returned to Virginia and started to research Alzheimer's on the Internet. There were medications now that could help in a limited way. To me, that meant that we needed to have her evaluated by a gerontologist. I talked with Mother and Dad and determined that I would set up an appointment for Mother in Lansing with a medical group associated with Michigan State University. Getting to Lansing was easier than getting to the University of Michigan in Ann Arbor.

I got all the ducks in a row and scheduled a trip to Michigan in October specifically for her doctor's appointment. Dad and I waited in the reception room. The tests were extensive. I guess that what I really wanted was a miracle, even though I wasn't aware of it at the time. The evidence was substantial, but still I wanted the assessment to be "not Alzheimer's."

The gerontologist joined us in the reception room. "Probable Alzheimer's," he said. When the words came out of his mouth, I felt like I had been slugged in the gut. Only then did I realize what I'd really hoped to hear. Despite all of my observations, I was wrong; it wasn't Alzheimer's. The thing to do now, the doctor continued, was to start planning for the future and how you as a family can care for her. Discuss medications with her and think about whether she wants to take them. Then, get back to us, he continued. No pressure. Time to let it all sink in.

A staff social worker mentioned adult day care, a new concept for me. The Lansing group knew about a well-established residential continuing care community, which had Alzheimer's programs, including day care, in a town near my parents' home. We talked about connecting with them.

"You may have to tell her that they want her to come help them as a volunteer," she said, opening the door just a crack to the way things might have to be framed in the future. Mother came back into the reception room. Her expression was naïve innocence. *Lamb to the slaughter*, I remembered thinking.

On the drive home, she told us she thought she had surprised "them" with how well she performed on the tests. My stomach turned as I considered her innocence and lack of reality.

As I went to bed that night on the living room sofa, the tears came and didn't stop. How in the world would I manage this from 700 miles away? My poor mother. My unresolved issues with her would remain unresolved. I would give her as much love as I could, because she was blood, my mother, and that's what I would want. My dad would be her primary caregiver. He would need all of the help I could give.

Yes, my life of independence would change.

My Stuff: Bandages Before Stitches

One of the reasons I had not picked up on my mother's early dementia/Alzheimer's symptoms in the early 1990s was the almost-breakdown I went through. I was in Philadelphia, falling apart at the seams. Years later I ended up being very grateful for the experience.

My fiftieth birthday was approaching. In a change of leadership, I had just been re-organized out of a job that I loved and did well. A significant flame from twenty years earlier had tracked me down with a guilt-ridden note. The woman he decided to marry instead of me appeared to be disappointing him. *Damn, what a shame,* I muttered under my breath.

Fortunately, I saw a skilled social worker/therapist during my meltdown.

Funny thing was I knew twenty years earlier that I would hear from Christopher, the old flame, again. I just didn't expect it to have the impact on me that it did. I had taken a temporary job that I was quickly learning to dislike. It was an exceptionally bad fit. I was depressed beyond description and aggressively pursuing my next job, wherever and whatever that would be.

I was a mess. I would look out the window of the suburban train taking me into Center City and tears would well up for no real reason. Serious depression. Oh, and once again I had not told my parents that I had lost my job. I told them when I got the new awful position, but not in the months before. My friends heard my agonies, but not my family.

Chris wanted to know all about my career since he was sure I was successful. I told him the truth, that I hadn't been successful in the traditional sense. If surviving was success, I had managed to pull that off, but that was it. Even though I looked younger than my age, it was clear to me that I was entering a dangerous time—too old to be hired at the price that I was worth, or, if I did get hired, I would be the first to go since I was expensive, especially with benefits and retirement plans.

I was too terrified to try going into my own business, largely because of the uncertainties my parents faced in theirs. Eventually I did form a limited liability partnership that worked well. But at the time it was more than I could wrap my head around. So, success was a word I almost gagged on.

Here, finally, was the letter that I knew would come someday. I guessed that I had a surprise or two to report to Chris. No, my life hadn't really worked out the way I might have hoped. Did he remember that I had wanted to have a child? I wrote back. I doubted that he had remembered. He had five children from his first marriage. "What was one more?" he'd told me at the time.

"You were my last chance to have a child," I wrote. But he saw me as *career woman*, whatever that meant to him. To me it meant more flexibility than it obviously did to him.

The women's movement, or the way the women's movement was interpreted at the time seemed to make these conversations more intense and harder to follow if you wanted a mix of family and career. Too many assumptions filled the gaps where inquiry and questions might have provided more authentic enlightenment. The timeframe for this conversation was between my twenty-ninth and thirty-third year.

My child-bearing equipment was also lousy, it turned out. At twenty-nine, I had major surgery designed to hold off a hysterectomy for a few years. Silly me, I didn't exactly hear the "few years" part. I should have listened more closely. Endometriosis and fibroid tumors were the official diagnoses. Not terribly unusual, but in a severe form that was potentially disabling for a career woman. So, yes, absolutely I would get that taken care of. I didn't spend enough time considering the other part of that issue: having a child. I just didn't seem to get the lesson on the biological clock. I was of the if-it-happens-it-happens school. *Not the smartest approach, but it didn't really register with me at the time.*

So, in my thirty-second or thirty-third year, things were challenging. Chris and I had broken off once again. "You're happy with things the way they are," he said.

"Well geez, I'm sorry," I replied.

He told me how much he wanted to be married again. The sad thing was it was the first I'd heard of it. This was the break-up conversation and here was new information. For the first time he told me he had been seeing a therapist. Apparently he and the therapist decided that I didn't want to be married and I was completely career-oriented. I pointed out that I should have been consulted on what I really wanted. But, I assumed that he and his therapist had made up their mind and he was not hearing my protests. So I gave up believing that he would eventually come to his senses and we'd try again. That's what we always did. *I didn't expect it to take twenty years, though.*

The next thing I knew he was planning to marry a woman who had one child. Yes, that got my attention and I probably spiraled into an undiagnosed depression. I moved on, but with unresolved sadness that I suppressed with job distractions and commitments. As the blues song says, "I still love you baby, but... I'm better off with the blues."[6]

My next jolt was my lousy reproductive equipment. In Michigan for Christmas, I started losing a lot of blood. I called the doctor's office from National Airport and went straight in. From there I went into minor surgery. I was told that there were no guarantees from here on out and that I could require emergency surgery the next time. So it was time to get things in order and schedule an elective procedure. I did, but I started to fall apart emotionally.

I descended into hell. Hormones added to the turmoil. I wanted to die but I was too much of a wimp to do anything about it. Though I wrote about these feelings in my journal, I don't know that I talked about them. Even when I found a helpful therapist, I was unable to work through my needs as a woman versus my career needs. The pragmatic me didn't have sufficient time to reach a comfort level with giving up on my desire to have a child. With the therapist, I put a bandage on the wound before I had stitches. And I really needed stitches. "Suck it up and move on," was the way I had learned to deal with my emotions, unfortunately.

Almost twenty years later, my losses erupted as post-traumatic-stress syndrome. I had suppressed the loss of the old flame and the loss of my ability to have children. Both of those blows occurred in the same timeframe. With the new loss of my job and turning fifty, I found myself in

---

6. Delbert McClinton, "Better Off With the Blues," by Delbert McClinton, Donnie Fritts, and Gary Nicholson, in *One of the Fortunate Few*, Curb (Universal), 1997, MP3.

a major depressive spiral. Fortunately, I was treated with medication and therapy. My therapist was trained in eye movement desensitization and reprocessing (EMDR), which worked for me. I also used antidepressants, which I continue to use today.

Though my mother could be a very depressed person, she didn't have the benefit of therapy and antidepressants. She wouldn't consider it—a generational thing perhaps. Research has strongly linked depression with vascular dementia and Alzheimer's.[7] Equally important, I would not have been equipped to handle Alzheimer's family caregiving without learning how to take care of my own mental health.

Yes, I had unresolved issues with my mother. I felt like I was expected to take care of her and respond like the adult from the age of twelve on. I promised my social worker/therapist before I left Philadelphia that I would continue therapy and work on my issues with my mother. Of course, I never got around to it in the way she intended.

---

7. Judith Graham, "Does Depression Contribute to Dementia?" *The New Old Age* (blog), *The New York Times*, May 1, 2013, http://newoldage.blogs.nytimes.com/2013/05/01/does-depression-contribute-to-dementia/?_r=0.

My Hometown

There it was: that long driveway to my 1960s house, still pretty forty years later. My trip from DC to St. Louis, Michigan had been easy. I turned right into the driveway.

"The other St. Louis," we used to explain, as we gave the address when I was a kid. The town was an interesting place, a community of three to four thousand in the 1950s. After World War II, workers from the south began to migrate to the more industrialized north. Mother and Dad were part of that migration, working at Michigan Chemical, the town's major employer.

It was a socially lively community with a population that valued education. There was a charming old hotel that was famous for its healing spa waters and duck dinners. I remembered, too, that the hotel was the site for a Valentine's Day party that was held before the Saturday Nighters' dance club. Mother and Dad were among the hosts.

In the 1960s, I used to brag that I "rode the school bus with Jim Northrup." He was the Detroit Tiger outfielder who hit a grand slam home run in the 1968 World Series. I always felt safe on the bus with any and all of the three Northrup boys. They were athletes and good guys. Sadly, Jim's obituary at age seventy-two said he had been in assisted living because of Alzheimer's disease.

The fifties and sixties were kind of the glory days for St. Louis. The little town had charm and a certain level of sophistication. Today, however, my hometown bears the scars of Michigan Chemical, later called Velsicol Chemical, which was the source of the pesticide DDT. The company saw one of the worst agricultural disasters in the country when polybrominated biphenyl (PBB), a fire retardant, entered the food chain in the early 1970s. Bags of the fire retardant were mixed with cattle feed by the Farm Bureau. More than 500 farms were quarantined, and thousands of beef cattle, sheep, swine, and chickens along with food products were destroyed.[8]

In an extensive environmental cleanup in 2012, the Environmental Protection Agency (EPA) returned to the St. Louis chemical plant site. That project, according to the *Detroit Free Press*, was the largest Superfund site in the six-state Great Lakes region. This cleanup was a continuation of one started nearly thirty years earlier. More than a $100 million has been spent, and dead robins were still found on lawns near the old plant site in 2014.

Thirty-five years earlier my father had a thyroid scare. We scheduled an appointment with endocrinologists at Johns Hopkins in Baltimore, MD. Dad went to the appointment, was asked where he lived. "It wouldn't be in the Saginaw Valley, would it?" the doctor asked.

"Why, yes." His thyroid problem was quickly diagnosed and treated with medication. The doctor said something about a high incidence of thyroid illnesses in that part of Michigan more than thirty years ago. His thyroid would come to haunt him in later years, too, as he developed Graves' disease. But there was never a way to easily trace possible causes and effects.

The 2010 census for St. Louis reported a phenomenal population increase of sixty-six percent in the ten years between census counts. I was stunned when I read it. That population increase, however, did not necessarily mean widespread economic vitality. It was likely that the increase from 4,494 to 7,482 came from the prison population, which had become a major employer. The city map listed three prisons. I guess the idea was that prison folks were permanent residents. Locals also said that families sometimes moved to St. Louis to be near their incarcerated family member. So despite the population increase, the glory days of cocktail parties and Saturday night dance clubs were long gone. So was trailer manufacturing in nearby Alma. Nearly all manufacturing businesses—chemicals, mobile homes (as the industry called them)—were gone.

Another memory. My high school debate partner went home from a

8. Michigan Department of Community Health, "PBBS (Polybrominated Biphenyls) in Michigan: Frequently Asked Questions—2011 Update," 1, https://www.michigan.gov/documents/mdch_PBB_FAQ_92051_7.pdf.

match we lost (we always lost) and murdered a young neighbor girl. Yes, murdered. So much for the goodness and safety of small towns. Worse yet, when the bone-chilling report came over the radio, I knew who might be responsible. The hair on the back of my neck stood straight up. I knew and to this day I don't know why I knew. I liked my partner, got along well with him, but he was a loner, isolated from other peers. Later press reports said he had carried a gun to school in his boot for several days. I think I got a letter from him after he was sent away. The letter seemed to disappear before I had a chance to answer it. I always suspected Mother or Dad was responsible for it vanishing. But, I can still remember that first news report. Whew!

Certainly it could be said that my feelings about my hometown were and are complicated, an odd mixture of pleasant and plainly gruesome memories. Awkward may be the best description. Like the sign in the park that described St. Louis: "This location marks the geographic center of the lower peninsula of Michigan AS CLOSELY AS CAN BE DETERMINED." Memorable in its awkwardness, that was my hometown. Not only did the sign in the park say that when i was a kid growing up, the website today still says that. Fortunately an editor appeared to get hold of more recent signage and boiled it down to the "center of the mitten." Progress.

Actually, we lived at the edge of St. Louis, a mile and a half from town. Typically i flew into lansing and rented a car. The house was home, but it was not where I grew up. I grew up in a trailer and a basement to a future dwelling next to the dry cleaners, four or five buildings west of this house. My mother and dad loved their new house. Me, not so much, even though it was well designed.

WHAT'S WRONG WITH MY FATHER?

In 2000, I had come home to take Mother to her doctor's appointment in Lansing. It had taken me from February to October to research gerontology specialists in Lansing, get the appointment, schedule a trip, and get home to begin the process of getting a formal diagnosis for Miss Dixie.

When my father walked through the garage to meet me, I was stunned. He had told me he didn't feel well and was losing weight for no reason. His shirt collar was so large it flapped. His face was drained of color. What's going on here?

"Doc's looking into it," Dad told me. Doc was Dr. James Hall, who was also a friend from Barbershoppers, Dad's singing group.

Suddenly it hit me that I had a bigger problem now. BOTH parents had serious health issues. This was getting complicated.

Then came our trip to Lansing to receive Mother's diagnosis. Despite a pile of evidence that dementia was under way, I carried the hope unknowingly that she would NOT have Alzheimer's. I was struck by how unprepared I was for the formal diagnosis. *First, her health. Now, his health, too. All of this—I really needed to get hold of it.* It looked like my focus would have to adjust from my mother's health to my father's. His problem was certainly more immediate, and the visuals said his health was the greater threat.

A month later, I went to a weekend silent retreat with friends from my meditation group. Thank heavens I came across this group in one of my Internet searches. As things progressed, meditation became a point of comfort, a tool to rid myself of thoughts and behavior that were counterproductive, and a solace beyond description.

I telephoned my dad. It was seven weeks since he started getting sick and one month since Mother's diagnosis. We searched back through any and everything that might have brought his health change on. The only major event we could think of was new dentures. All Kincaids have lousy teeth, including me. He had had dentures so long I don't remember him with anything else. And when I looked at pictures from his early years, his teeth never showed. Sometimes there was a smile, but it was a smile with no teeth showing. His new dentures were ugly and fit badly, but not so much as to cause his mysterious weight loss.

Dad's latest test was for his heart. He had not been feeling well the last two days. The cardiologist told him he had the heart of a 48-year-old. Dad was clearly pleased, but the mystery continued. He had always been incredibly fit and free of chronic health problems. As a 78-year-old man, he was hopping around on the roof of our commercial building directing its redesign and rebuilding. Healthy and energetic. The opposite of Mother, who had headaches, back aches, and various pains all her adult life.

"How's Mother doing?" I asked.

"She's just great," he reported. *Just great?* "She's watering her plants and taking the dead leaves away." The tone of his voice and his words reflected the man of optimism I had always known. *He's back,* I thought to myself.

Doc was systematically ruling out potential causes. He started with cancer. Clear. Then, his heart. Clear. When the heart was ruled out, the next step was finding an endocrinologist. The first appointment with one was two months away. After an Internet search and a review of another specialist's *curriculum vitae,* I telephoned and was able to get an appointment in two weeks.

The specialists were in Lansing. I was 700 miles away. Who would drive my father? It turned out Dad's friends from Barbershoppers would. Team Kincaid was beginning to form. "The guys," as Dad called them, took care of his transportation issues. He could no longer see well enough to drive himself safely.

Ray Anspaugh was the grocery guy and my dad's golf partner. Grant Colthorp took him to the doctor when he could and looked in on him regularly. Grant and Dad met when Grant was a scrawny teenager looking for a job. He got the position, along with a lifelong close friendship and a bond resembling a father/son relationship. Ken Smith, who had taught science at an area community college, connected Dad with a former student who was an optometrist and drove Dad to doctor's appointments. And Jim "Doc" Hall, Dad's primary care physician, would even drive him to Lansing for medical appointments if no one else was available. They were the Fab Four forever and always. They made sure the important things were covered.

As for Mother? Her health situation had been moved rather abruptly to the back burner.

A couple of weeks later and it was Thanksgiving. For the first time in years, I spent the holiday with Mother and Dad. I began a pattern that would carry on for the next few years and would become one of my favorite memories to look back on. I'd leave my house in Arlington at 6:30 a.m. on Thanksgiving Day. Arrive in Detroit at 9:30. Connect with a flight to Lansing or rent a car and drive on home. This time I couldn't find a connecting flight that would get me home in time to cook Thanksgiving dinner. So, I rented a car in Detroit and drove the two and a half hours to St. Louis.

I stopped in Okemos at a grocery store and picked up a small fresh turkey, frozen peas, fresh parsley and onions, butter, etc. I was carrying frozen cranberry relish and carrot soup that I made earlier. Thanksgiving dinner in a flash and it was good!

"Good to have you home, honey," my frail-looking father told me as I started dinner. Despite his bad health, Dad had peeled potatoes immersed in water, waiting to be cooked. So that job was done. A couple of days before, Dad had his appointment with the endocrinologist in Lansing. Doc drove, my dad told me, and Ken Smith had stopped by and was sitting in the living room as backup in case Doc had scheduled himself too tightly. Doc made the trip and was asked by the endocrinologist how he happened to be with his patient.

"He's a friend and a Barbershopper," Doc replied, as though there was nothing unusual about the trip. "The Dream Team" in action.

Even though our health focus was on Dad, I was weighing and measuring the changes in my mother, too. People she loved, she could no longer remember. I kept doing what I should not have done by trying to feed her clues to help her memory. Dumb and frustrating for her and me.

Then, I screwed up my courage and asked the question eating away at me.

"Did Grandmother know who you were?" I asked. Mother used to say that the most important thing she did was to be with her mother and father when they died as she and Lucille, her sister and life-long best friend, cared for them.

"It was the reflection in her face," my mother replied, avoiding a direct response. "That was so beautiful. The look in her eyes..." I took that to be a "no." It made me sad and I didn't understand why it was so important to me. *Get over it,* I said to myself.

Years later I could still replay the scene. We were sitting in the living room of the Michigan house. Outside the ground was crunchy from snow and the cold temperature. At this point, she knew she had Alzheimer's and talked about it without fear. I even asked her, "Are you afraid?"

"No," she said, "because of Mother. There are so many things that could be worse. Cancer..."

My mother's acceptance appeared to be unusual. No bitterness. In fact, her acceptance without sorrow was the only one I ever heard of. I don't ever remember hearing acceptance without anger or sorrow as a response in more than ten years with caregiving support groups. My mother embraced her new reality without bitterness, despair, or denial. I often wondered if I would be able to do the same when my turn came. I doubted it.

At this point, she was accepting her diagnosis better than I was. We had stopped to get some plants for the living room while we were in Mt. Pleasant.

"This is where I notice my disease," she said with remarkable awareness. "I used to be able to imagine, to see what it might look like at home. Now, I can't." My mother, the painter, the visual communicator, recognized things were beginning to change. Then she told me an ugly pair of snow boots looked "cute" and I bought them.

As Mother and I were having our evening conversation she told me, "I think of you every night before I go to sleep." Shocked and touched, I was a basket case when she said that. Here was a woman fighting to remember as long as she could because she understood how important it was to me. That would change for me later, but then I really felt it was important.

I fell asleep on the sofa and woke to see her covering me up. Later, she slept fitfully in a lounge chair in the family room. A blood-curdling scream interrupted the night at some point, and then a soft voice said, "I'm sorry."

A tear trickled down my face to my pillow before I fell back asleep. So much going on.

Articulated throughout my journal was my fear. *Am I beginning to get Alzheimer's now? If not now, when?* The ongoing angst of being a child of Alzheimer's. Not the most important thing I had to deal with, but underlying each day and decision when things quieted down and I started to write.

CHRISTMAS 2000

In no time at all, it was Christmas. From 700 miles away I scheduled a doctor's appointment for Dad so that I could go with him, an appointment later in the day for Mother in Lansing, and, later in the week, time to see rooms at the Masonic Home in Alma and learn about their Alzheimer's day care program.

I arrived after an icy beautiful snow. I made the first of many mistakes by providing too much information. I told Mother we needed to plan what she was going to wear to the doctor's appointment in the afternoon.

Over and over. "What am I going to wear? Why are we going?" Too much information was a mistake, I eventually taught myself. But, in the early years I had to learn it the hard way. We left Mother at home while I took Dad to his appointment. Doc re-capped: fifty pounds lost in a matter of four months, no cancer that we have been able to find, and his thyroid functioning at a pace that was seven times what it should be. Eventually the diagnosis was Graves' disease, and Dad's bulging eyes crowded the optic nerve, nearly blinding him.

As we went home to take Mother to Lansing, fifty miles away, for her appointment, I found her in the bathroom with blood all over. A dark spot on a varicose vein had popped and the bathroom looked like a television murder scene. Cancel the Lansing appointment. We called Doc to see if he could work her in and help get the bleeding stopped. Instead, he came to the house so that we didn't have to take her to the emergency room. Later that evening, my dad looked at me with a twinkle in his eye.

"Next time we'll put the bandages on her the night before," he said. Our learning curve on managing explanations to our Alzheimer's patient needed some work. I laughed and agreed.

I started making soup—one of my favorite therapeutic approaches and also a useful one, since filling the freezer was one of my self-determined responsibilities while I was home each time. One year my dad had me make carrot soup for the Fab Four and we took freezer packages around at Christmastime with a holiday note of thanks. Dad had taken over the cooking responsibilities and was already managing her medications, handing them to her and watching her take them.

My visit to the Masonic Home in Alma was an opportunity to learn about day care programs for Alzheimer's patients. It was an informative visit and it also included the residential options. I showed Mother the floor plans and she was excited by the possibilities, but that didn't last long.

Other financial matters needed attention. A couple of years earlier we had done the wills, powers of attorney, and medical power of attorney for Michigan. But Mother had still been trying to keep the books and pay bills. She was adamant that my father not do it. "You won't do it right," she yelled at him and me. I would do it, I told her.

It was an awful night of yelling and screaming. Eventually, World War III settled down and I started transferring their checkbook details to my bookkeeping software. After this sad confrontation, which included moments of rationality, she admitted that trying to keep the checkbook straight gave her a headache. I wondered how long it had been giving her a headache and how long she had tried to carry on.

At two in the morning, I woke to see the lights on and hear papers rustling. The tables in the dining room and a card table in the living room were archeological digs of old receipts and bank statements. Piles of papers were covered by white sheets, my mother's solution to the visual assaults of clutter. There was also hoarding. Indeed, the hallway to the second bathroom was barely passable. It was filled with furniture pieces acquired, no doubt, at a wonderful price at some auction sale. For what and for whom? *Never mind.*

Then there was paper. In Miss Dixie's bookkeeping system, the years of telephone, utility receipts, and bank statements were layered, more or less. A year or two was covered by the white bed sheet. Then, another year or two of useless paper was covered by another white bed sheet. So, part of my trips home included "sort and shred" as well as clearing out the furniture in the hallway so that the hallway was passable, more or less. In the paper sorting, sometimes Mother would sit beside me while I worked, and sometimes she was completely uninterested. When she looked at the pieces of paper now, her disease prevented her from understanding what they meant, so she just left them.

A secondary objective of sort and shred was looking for missing cash. At least $500 was gone, according to my dad. One evening Mother and I were doing one of the layers of the card table set up in the living room when her hand shot out quickly. I had not seen them yet. She laid out two $100 bills.

She turned to me, leaned in, and whispered. "I'll split it with you." I laughed out loud. We never found the other $300, or the beautiful antique earrings I got her for her eightieth birthday (which I especially wanted). Just disappeared.

As I became more involved with the finances, I was shocked by the number of companies that tried to bully old people into buying stuff they didn't need. It ranged from credit cards to books that kicked in if the individual did not explicitly respond "no." What was a blind man, my father, going to do with books from Reader's Digest? When I wrote to remove his name from the mailing list, I said:

"He is nearly blind and eighty-five years old. I find it hard to believe that he has ordered the books you are charging him with...

"Any future bullying about payment will be viewed as a hostile action and I will proceed to draw as much public attention as possible to your outrageous sales tactics among older, disabled people to state attorneys general."

Then there was Master Card, where the annual fee kicked in automatically and grew monthly if left unpaid. Mother neither asked for nor needed a Master Card account. I saw her hands shake as she brought this bill to my attention. She was frightened and terribly confused by these nasty con games; older people are so at risk for the unscrupulous. Disgusting and appalling. I enjoyed canceling accounts and settling scores to some extent with these SOBs.

Toward the end of my stay, it happened. My mother didn't know who I was for the first time, and I learned it wasn't such a big deal after all.

*

In all of the concern about Dad's health, I had failed to move ahead with the one medication that had been recommended to Mother at the time of her diagnosis. So, I asked her.

"Do you want to try the medication?"

"Yes, of course," she said, and we got her prescription going. My dad, the thrifty Scotsman, had a fit over the price. Something like $4 a pill at the time. *Welcome to one of the early costs of Alzheimer's*, I thought. (Generics are now available on the first basic medications.)

Nonetheless, the Scotsman parted with significant cash for a fancy adjustable bed. Mother talked about how well she slept in it. Her miserable sleeping habits of more than a decade suddenly improved. Did the sleep improvement help slow her dementia? I couldn't tell. Sleep problems have begun to show up as a characteristic in some Alzheimer's research.[9]

In this early phase of Alzheimer's, things were happening, but happening slowly. One of her first symptoms had been judgment and reasoning, and then the more conspicuous memory loss with the repetition of questions. That was followed by a decline in language skills. She was simply unable to find the right word. I also noticed new words coming into her vocabulary. "Cross" as a description of behavior toward her, usually my father's. "Yum," "sniffles," and "blabbering" were new words that I came to hear. She had always used the word "chatter" to describe words she didn't particularly want to hear.

She explained to me that she no longer asked people what they meant unless she knew them really well. I had to smile because I have done that all of my life.

Her conversational capacity was changing. She had always loved the telephone, but was already beginning to shy away from it. Her experience on this issue came much earlier than many Alzheimer's patients I have heard about in my caregivers support group. In addition, one of the things I worried in my journal about was whether I was still giving her the respect she deserved as my mother. This was my first formal recognition that roles were changing.

Researching Alzheimer's on the National Institute on Aging webpage

9. "Poor Sleep May Be Linked to Alzheimer's Disease," ALZinfo.org, reviewed by William J. Netzer, PhD, https://www.alzinfo.org/articles/poor-sleep-may-be-linked-to-alzheimers-disease/.

was taking an increasing amount of my time. I also found a caregivers support group, led by a wonderful geriatric nurse who had taken some time off to unwind after an intense professional assignment. The group lost her when she decided she needed to focus on one volunteer activity, but her guidance set a high standard for information on the disease.

I'm sure this was where I was introduced to the Activities of Daily Living (ADLs, since everything in the healthcare field must be reduced to an incomprehensible acronym). The activities are bathing, dressing, toileting, eating, and "mobility issues," such as walking and getting in and out of a chair or bed independently. How many of these skills the patient still retains suggests where he or she is in the progression of Alzheimer's disease. They also serve as placement guides for day care, assisted living, skilled nursing care, etc.

A Moment of Grace and Clarity

Still grappling and struggling with how I felt about the road ahead, I encountered a moment of inspiration and clarity. I have since come to characterize it as a moment of grace.

Spring flowers were blooming, and it was a beautiful day. I was attending a meditation weekend seminar and sitting outside during a lunch break with a woman I knew slightly. "It really isn't that bad," she commented. Caring for someone with Alzheimer's is *really not that bad.* I was stunned, and I would look back on this conversation as a monumental shift in the way I viewed Alzheimer's and my role as a caregiver. At the time, all I had heard was how awful and dreadful it was taking care of someone with dementia. Here was someone who had helped her father through his last days, saying it really wasn't all that bad.

"My brother handled it better than I did," she continued. "He was more laid back about what was going on, and I was trying to structure too much." Her comments were astonishing. That insight happened within months of my mother's diagnosis of dementia/probable Alzheimer's. Up until that point, I had been all weepy. Suddenly there was a bit of a light, and the way I saw my future as an Alzheimer's caregiver changed dramatically. Don't assume disaster. There may be some bright spots.

When I thought back, it did seem Mother's dark side was diminished. She was happy and cheerful—not consumed by depression and sadness. She was loopy, but sweet and pleasant to be around generally. She was not the angry patient to be feared. Nonetheless, she could be exceedingly difficult.

Personal hygiene became an enormous issue for my dad. "She won't take a shower," he would report on the phone. When I got back to Michigan, she smelled really bad. Unbelievable, given her practices before

Alzheimer's. We tried unsuccessfully to talk her into getting a shower. From time to time our cajoling would head into scolding. Absolutely the wrong approach. Once, when we were still trying to get her to do it by herself, she turned to Dad and me and said: "I want you two to tell each other how much you LIKE me." Smiling sweetly, she made her exit, stage left. Dad and I laughed. How could you not?

Miss Dixie's charm was taking a new turn. The tough stuff could be balanced on our memory cards with moments of joy and humor.

Each trip back to Michigan, I would schedule medical and dental appointments for Mother and Dad. At one of these, the technician was going on and on about stuff I had trouble following. The moment the tech left earshot, Miss Dixie turned to me: "That didn't do a thing for me. How about you?"

An Unexpected Trip to West Virginia

Just as winter was settling in, I answered the phone to hear my father report that Uncle Loman's wife had died. Loman was one of my mother's younger brothers. He had also been a partner in the dry cleaning business with Mother and Dad for a while. "Would you come home and drive us to West Virginia for the funeral?" "Let me see what I can do," I replied. Ordinarily, my scheduled trips were every six weeks. Since I was also self-employed as a consultant, I had a moderately flexible work schedule. For this unscheduled trip, I managed to pick up a more-expensive-than-usual ticket to Detroit and went on home.

When I arrived to prepare for this West Virginia road trip, I found Mother's hair in a state of disarray. So, that's when I started cutting and styling her hair. I did a decent job. She looked pretty good, and doing it was very satisfying to me for some reason. When I cut and styled her hair on a later trip, she reached for her purse to pay me. "No, not necessary," I said, smiling.

At that point Mother had lost about forty of the eighty or so pounds that she eventually lost. I had sent her a black jacket earlier, just so she would have something to wear given her weight loss. We loaded the car and headed to West Virginia. Mother and Loman had always been close. She walked in his house and, despite her Alzheimer's, immediately became his older, take-charge sister.

"You need a haircut," she announced. "Well, I've been taking care of Madelyn and didn't have time to get one," he replied. Uncle Loman, according to us cousins, had the habit of showing up in $1,000 suits. He used to tell me his suits weren't really that expensive, but I'm not sure I believed him. He knew fabric and he almost always had an elegant navy blue suit or blazer on, along with a great tie and beautiful shirt.

"Sit down," my mother ordered. Despite the fact that he was all dressed for the wake, she was determined to get his hair and collar line straightened out. Out came the scissors and she went to work. She was slow, and he grumbled that she was going to take an ear off, but she did a remarkably good job.

On this trip, I took a picture of Mother and Dad with the Ohio River in the background standing arm in arm, and it is one of my favorites. The leaves were off the trees, so it could have been a stark backdrop, but I never felt that way about it. It was simply a different view of their homeland, and a view without West Virginia's mountains. I also remembered two young women turning to look at my octogenarian parents walking arm in arm through a restaurant and whispering how sweet they looked. Dad was probably wearing one of his brother's hand-me-down suits. After the service, I heard my mother say, "I have Alzheimer's don't you know." Sweetly, happily... a simple matter of fact.

*

In 2001, I had already planned to take Mother and Dad to West Virginia for Christmas. I flew home at Christmas time intent on spending it in West Virginia, since everyone was able this year and who knew what the future would bring. My recently widowed aunt was going through her second Christmas without my father's oldest brother, and we were looking forward to being with her. Dad's health was still a challenge. His vision was gone because of Graves' disease. We had been back and forth to Lansing for his eyes, and to an endocrinologist.

The Graves' disease was beginning to settle down, but his eyesight was not improving. He was depressed over it, understandably. It seemed that the optic nerve was crowded by the Graves', and he would likely need surgery at the beginning of next year to cut away the bone.

Off we went to West Virginia for a visit to Dad's remaining siblings and my mother's nieces. Cousin Candace had Christmas dinner for any and all. Children, spouses, sister, grandchildren, neighbors, and us. Just like the reunions Granddad and Grandmother had at the farm. That was the first time I met Candace's grandchildren, and I was touched to see a young granddaughter named Lucille, named for her late great grandmother and my mother's sister. It was an unexpected reminder of the family legacy.

On the way somewhere, Dad wanted to drive through Charleston.

His college, Morris Harvey, had been absorbed and re-named the University of Charleston.

We drove along the Kanawha River as Dad pointed out from the front passenger seat where he'd lived, as well as the hilltop that he and Mother had visited when they were dating. "Mother, that's where we used to go to spoon," he said.

Suddenly a little voice piped up from the back seat.

"Wasn't me. Must've been some other woman," Miss Dixie, the jokester, said, looking out the side window. In the rear mirror, I could see a slight smile and sparkle in her eye.

The Garretts of Looneyville, West Virginia

That trip to West Virginia was far different from the one I first remembered as a child. Michigan to West Virginia was my first big road trip. Our destination: Looneyville, West Virginia. *Yes, I know.*

"Daddy, stop it," my four-year-old self cried from the back seat of that black 1940s Ford. "You make me fall." The car rolled from one side to the other, rounding the twisting curves of the mountain roads.

Since he always read the Sunday comics to me, I was sure he would listen. It was HIS driving, I knew. I blamed my father loudly. I was pitched from one side of the back seat to the other long before there were safety seats for children. I had learned to ride in the car in Michigan, where the roads were straight and the land flat. He drove the narrow roads and curving hills of West Virginia at a reasonable speed. My father laughed, refused to straighten his driving up because he couldn't, and I took it personally.

My maternal grandparents lived miles from a community of any size—Spencer, which was also the county seat for Roane County. The scenery was stunning, except for the blemishes of devastating poverty, still present today. Green trees up and down the hills. Narrow two-way roads. Rust-colored rocks in streaks and layers on one side, and precarious drops on the other. The cliff-like drops when I looked out the window seemed to go forever. Every now and then there was a small stretch that was sort of straight enough for passing, but I don't remember that we ever passed anyone.

Those roads were nothing compared to the rock-based back road of half a mile that connected the Garrett family farm with the main road. Imagine several hundred speed bumps strung together and that was the feel in that little black Ford crawling its way to Grandmother and Granddad's house. At the curve just before you could see the Garrett house was the long winding driveway that led to Lucille's house. Lucille was my mother's older sister.

My grandmother was about my mother's height, five feet six inches. She always wore dresses and aprons. Her long gray hair was pulled back into a twisted bun, and her shoes were sensible laced-up black things with a relatively low heel. At least her dress shoes looked like that. Sometimes she wore worn-out men's shoes around the house. The other family members were extremely tall. Granddad was well over six feet, as were Lucille and her five brothers. Another sister, Lenore, whom I remember seeing a few times in childhood, was maybe five feet eight or so. Lucille was eighteen months older than my mother, Dixie. Lucille was fourth in birth order and Dixie, fifth. Growing up, Dixie was close to Lenore. Lenore taught her how to sew; Lucille didn't care one whit about sewing. Lenore married young, while Lucille and Mother married in their twenties. Lucille and Dixie were best friends forever, despite different temperaments. They and several other siblings also shared a love of antiques, with a competitive edge in their respective collections.

Eight relatively tall children, one very tall father and a medium-sized mother came from a house that was probably twenty feet wide at most. It was small and rickety. The house had one bedroom with two large beds, no bathroom, a kitchen, a dining room, and a living room that had a double bed, in addition to a sleeper sofa. I remembered its gray, weathered-board exterior, later covered by green shingles (asbestos no doubt) in a home improvement ordered and executed by my mother as Mountaineer Tiger Project Manager. Just outside the kitchen door was a hand pump, which contained the drinkable water from a well. All other water came from runoff from the various farm buildings that went into a cistern for non-potable water. There was a cellar outbuilding that contained all of the home canning from the garden and farm. Crocks of sauerkraut fermenting. Canned meat from the fall slaughter. Canned tomatoes and green beans from the garden.

On top of the cellar was a sleeping annex probably first built for the boys—the five brothers. Later, it was used by visiting grandchildren when we got old enough to be trusted on our own. Then there was the washhouse. A toilet that flushed sometimes, especially if there was enough rain for water pressure, a shower, a sink, a wringer laundry machine, and some indoor clotheslines for drying towels and clothes.

The small, weary house sat on cement blocks. Under the house became a favorite place for cats and dogs, not to mention the occasional errant chicken. The floors were drafty in winter, but, since free natural gas was one of the few perks for farm landowners, no one worried that much about winter heating bills. Big natural gas heaters pumped warmth into the dining and living rooms. The dining room heater was a gathering spot for farm men after supper.

The view from under the shade tree was spectacular. It was the top of our ridge and it looked out across rolling hills, green and lush in the summer, glorious red and gold in the fall when the trees in the distance began to turn.

Even though there was a large wooden box telephone at Grandmother's, it was never clear what the phone was connected to. The wall phone held a prominent place, right by the front door. I heard stories that it was a party line that went nowhere. Not to town, certainly. We couldn't call in from the outside world. More often than not, Lucille and Grandmother would yell across the hollow to one another. I don't remember at all what their code was, but it seemed to work, since Lucille often showed up with a perfectly splendid coconut cake not long after.

By far the most spectacular meal of the day to my visiting eyes was breakfast. Killer homemade biscuits every morning. We grandchildren used to beg for a recipe, only to be greeted by a smile and a report of a little of this, more of that, etc. Grandmother never used anything written on paper. I don't remember that our mothers ever uncovered the secret, nor did we grandchildren. As for the rest of the menu: creamed tomatoes, some sweetened canned apples or applesauce (homemade, of course), homemade sausage and eggs, and potatoes. There was nothing like the smell and taste of an early morning breakfast on the farm.

The refrigerator was in the dining room. There was usually a churn somewhere in the dining room, too. After breakfast, Grandmother worked the churn. I remember when an electric churn was greeted as an important labor-saving device. As a short little kid, I got to sit back next to the wall and the window with its lacey curtains. I liked my spot because I could watch the outside and inside inconspicuously. Forever the observer... *Euwwoo, I just saw my grandmother twirl a chicken around by its neck. Til it died. Sunday dinner. Don't think I'm going to watch the rest.*

Across the dining room I remember a very long picture, maybe three feet long, of soldiers all standing in line outside a military barracks. My Uncle Loman was the only one I could identify. As I grew older, I came to notice a similarity in height among all the soldiers in this very long line. The famous four-star General George S. Patton seemed to take a liking to young Appalachian men with a similar hardy look. Probably just legend, but I came to like it as an explanation. Uncle Loman was a part of Patton's march through Africa and Germany, including the Battle of the Bulge. Only later as an adult did I realize the significance of his World War II service.

Individual photos topped a good-sized chest of drawers next to the refrigerator. Uncle Richard, another World War II star, was there looking dashing in his Air Force pilot's gear. What a handsome man. My tall, gorgeous uncles. On top of the lace doily were more pictures. Cousins who were older and who I rarely saw were there, along with cousins who were my age: sisters Candace and Kate, Karen Sue, and sometimes me, Barbara Kay. The famous Garrett smiles were there: Uncle Herbert, who I never remember having hair, but whose fabulous, welcoming smile I will never forget. He was the smart, reliable older brother. Gardner extraordinaire. Mr. Wonderful.

Candace and Kate were Lucille's daughters. Lucille, like Herbert, was an educator. Herbert was an elementary school principal for many years, but Lucille taught forty years in country schools, many of which were one room with all eight grades. She was country smart, with real street cred along Vineyard Gap and Clover, where she taught. Though I had known Lucille all of my early life, I got to know her better when she came to Baltimore and Uncle Herbert's house for treatment from Johns Hopkins.

Then there was Grandmother Losa, the only grandmother I ever knew. She was also the first in my family who was known to have Alzheimer's. My view of my grandmother has changed. Based on observations from my cousins who lived close by, I am now convinced I had her all wrong. I saw her as sweet, quiet, and perfect. I still think of her as perfect, but a lot more interesting as a personality than I witnessed in my summer trips to West Virginia. Sweet and soft spoken, yes. But some sharp vinegar in there, too. A Mountaineer Tiger Woman resided behind that sweet façade. I didn't even know it until my mother was gone. I always wondered. My mother had fire and looked like my grandmother.

And Miss Dixie saw herself as like her mother. But, I never understood how alike they were until both were gone. Although Granddad had diabetes and a range of health issues Grandmother, as she aged, seemed to have two: a bad back and Alzheimer's.

Granddad had stomach surgery in his sixties. After, he lost a lot of weight, easily eighty to a hundred pounds. Yet he was still a big man. Grandmother called him Ed, shortened from Loman Edgar. His sons liked to call him "Lij," short for Elijah, the 9th century B.C. Hebrew prophet, and a name generally synonymous with strength. While the origin of the nickname was uncertain, I always figured it had something to do with his physical presence. Small boys, probably his own children, decided at an early age that his height, weight, and general presence merited the name. Imposing: that's what I remembered.

I saw Grandmother as this incredibly competent homemaker who cooked, sewed, and took care of her garden—a massive thing that sustained a family of ten and various farm hands who dropped by. Gentle and kind. She was all of those things in her Alzheimer's as well.

Grandmother also taught her children good manners and reading if they happened to be struggling in school. Loman, her sixth child, did struggle. Every night he sat in the kitchen while Grandmother fixed supper and read to her, spelling the words to her as he tried to learn them. Soon his reading was where it should be.

Once, when I was visiting without my parents, she let it slip that my grandfather drank; something my mother would have denied if I had asked her. Fortunately I was wise enough at the age of ten not to ask. By the way, legend has it that Granddad, a Southern Democrat, was so angry with the election of President Dwight D. Eisenhower in 1952 that he QUIT drinking. Some woman in a bar was celebrating her candidate's victory and hassling my granddad about it so much that he went off the sauce completely. Personally, I've never known an election to be a reason to sober up, but apparently '52 was for my grandfather.

For all her kindness, my grandmother was a woman not to be messed with. This never occurred to me, since I remembered her sweet, soft laugh and her welcoming call to neighbors who were just passing by. However, stories have emerged. Grandmother was not afraid to act. Smart, but without a lot in the way of formal education, her own mother died at the age of thirty-nine. Losa was ten when she started taking care of her two brothers and a sister, Lydia, who was blind and pretty much a rattlesnake on a good day. Losa's mother and father were first cousins, both Vineyards, and that inter-marriage created health issues. Grandmother had a conspicuously curved spine, though I don't remember the direction of the curve now. Mostly, I remember that it didn't look comfortable.

Grandmother and Granddad were nineteen when they married, and their eight children started arriving in 1910, with roughly eighteen months between each child. But family stories suggest that, in addition to the old booze issue, my dear grandfather might have had a wandering eye. At home and extremely busy, Grandmother still was not to be fooled. She had a way of figuring out what was going on and who her competition might be.

One evening she had Herbert, her second-oldest son, babysit the younger children while she went to visit her competition's household. She walked down the road through the pasture of the neighboring farm. It would not have been an easy jaunt. Especially not with a shotgun. Yes, Sweet Losa was packing heat. When the competition's door opened, Grandmother raised the shotgun to her shoulder and tried to blow the big wooden phone box off the wall. She was marginally successful. The Mountaineer Tiger Woman had made her point.

It took some effort from Granddad to keep folks from prosecuting Sweet Losa. The victims were understandably annoyed and took it personally, which is, of course, what Grandmother had in mind, and they took to carrying the phone box on its piece of wall around as evidence. Granddad paid. It's not clear whether there was a conversation between Grandmother and Granddad about events or not. Grandmother might have had a lot of sewing to do or chickens to kill.

Apparently, Granddad did not significantly change his ways. Another competitor was known to be superstitious. She had a pattern of walking through the hills and meeting Granddad in the field just as the moon came up at night. One clear, crisp fall evening something rather amazing happened: a ghost appeared. From behind a huge mound of hay. All white and scary. Superstitious and terrified, the woman shrieked her way home, stayed home, and presumably lost interest in fooling around with Ed Garrett. No longer a problem. Grandmother could make a rug from old rags or a ghost from a sheet.

To his credit, Granddad worried if his many granddaughters would think less of him when his early traveling ways came to light. We didn't. In fact, we were mostly fascinated by the strength of Grandmother's response. Kind of a "you go girl" thing. Of course Dixie, my dear mother, would have denied that it ever happened. Her father fool around? No, NEVER!

Losa also demonstrated her strong will and resolve in other ways. Education was a familiar theme. She and her brother joined forces to use some Vineyard family land for an early one-room schoolhouse where her children and nieces and nephews were taught. When it was time for Herbert to enroll in college, Grandmother wrote the tuition check. Then, after the fact, she told Granddad. He was forced to sell some cattle quickly to cover the check. A shrug of the shoulders and a smile was likely her explanation. Herbert had potential and she knew it. His education was not a matter to be debated.

My mother's stories of hard times during the Depression were compelling. She described a level of poverty that I had trouble imagining. Food was scarce, but there was still the garden, so the impact was less dire than in the cities. At the same time, there was no extra income from trading and selling livestock. Dirt poor. Play clothes? No, only the clothes on your back. My mother remembered being forced to hide naked behind the hill while her only dress was washed and dried. As an adult, my mother had to have things—attractive clothes, good linens, sterling silver—perhaps as a result of this early deprivation.

Then came the war, and concern shifted to the survival of three sons in World War II. Each returned without a scratch, despite serving in heavy combat. Marriages, grandchildren. Ups and downs and suddenly Grandmother and Granddad were no longer able to handle the hands-on labor of the farm and farm life. But that was okay. The world was changing. Grocery stores replaced gardens. And, Alzheimer's moved in.

FAMILIES CARE FOR EACH OTHER

When did I become so hooked on my extended family? I think it was when I was a child. Somewhere, too, a "rule" was hardwired in my brain: families care for each other. Certainly I was hooked on both my maternal and paternal families. They were fun, a little bit crazy, and interesting. I knew this even as a kid. Was it because my family of origin was so small? Maybe. There wasn't anything I could do about it. My mother lost a second child and the capacity to bear future children when I was almost three. An ectopic fallopian tube pregnancy.

I remembered visiting her in the hospital. I stood on some steps so I could reach her hospital bed. I had been a brat and complained loudly. "Aunt Naudie spank me," I reported. I had been staying with my mother's older brother, Herbert, and his wife Maudie (Maude) in Spencer. I think my mother was in the hospital in Charleston, so it would have been a big deal to take me to the hospital, fifty miles away on bumpy, curving state roads. There were no interstate highways in those days.

My mother was unsympathetic. I got spanked because I hid under the dining room table where my very pregnant four-foot-ten-inch aunt could not reach me. Clearly, I had figured out my advantage. As she circled the table, I could keep myself just out of her arm's reach. I didn't want to take a nap. Eventually, she got hold of me, though. There might have been a cookie involved, and the brat was spanked. I was extremely disappointed that my mother refused to take my side and support my claim of abuse.

Eventually, Aunt Naudie and I became great friends. She, Uncle Herbert, and Aunt Lucille were very important characters in my adult life. By the time my career took me to Washington, Uncle Herbert and Aunt Maude were living outside of Baltimore. I stayed with them for a year while I was trying to renovate the lower level of a little house I bought on a creek near the Chesapeake Bay, just north of Annapolis, Maryland. Even after I got settled in Severna Park, I used to meander up on a Saturday and sit around the kitchen table talking about family stories and legends. The Baltimore Garretts were smart, sensible, and caring, and I was not connected with or enchanted by Washington in the early years. I was a little lonely, to be perfectly honest.

They lived on several acres in a wonderful farmhouse that they had taken from disaster to a charming and lovely family residence, filled with their various collections of antiques. Springtime at their house was stunning. Thousands of daffodils lined the large side yard along the country road. Then there were flowering trees: cherry, apple, peach, and pear. In the kitchen, there was a wonderful old oak sideboard and the shelves were loaded with old pieces of pewter. We sat at a round oak table sipping tea, and I listened to stories and reports on other family members in West Virginia.

The Baltimore Garretts had almost fallen off the family map a couple of years before. Lydia Vineyard, who was Grandmother Garrett's blind sister, had shown up on their doorstep. She was old, probably poor, bitter, and not known for a pleasant personality in the best of times. I never met her and knew her only by legend. My mother said she was mean. She wasn't born blind, but there was some kind of childhood accident that might have involved my grandmother, so she spent most of her life angry. Nonetheless, on that busy West Virginia farm on Vineyard Ridge, Aunt Lydia took pity on Herbert. A third grader, he was struggling to learn how to read when Aunt Lydia pulled him out of the chaos of his siblings and cousins, sat him under a tree, and taught him. Garretts were loyal and had long memories. He certainly used that reading, too, since he ended up as the Garrett with the most education, all-but-a-doctoral dissertation from Johns Hopkins University. There was always a special bond between Aunt Lydia and Herbert. She kept in touch with no one else in the family, just Herbert. So, when she needed help, Herbert was the one she turned to.

Not only was he to help her, but she also demanded he tell no one else in the family that she was with them. Or about her condition, which Aunt Maude said was horrific. Lydia had a facial cancer that was disfiguring. A vile, untreatable disfigurement that also had a disturbing smell, according to my aunt. Lydia's care was extremely difficult. Lots of complaining and yelling was a part of her misery. There might have been some Alzheimer's in there, too. Who knows?

Eventually, the Baltimore Garretts were able to get her into a long-term care facility, but there was a long wait—at least a year for admission. The two Garrett daughters, Nancy and Jane Ann, were the only ones who knew about the secret resident in Baltimore. They were told not to come home while she was in the house. Silence to the other family members was the order of the day. Dixie was sure something was wrong. She pushed and prodded, but could never pin it down. After Lydia died and was buried in Baltimore, the story came out. So, that set the framework for one caregiving example in my extended family. You took care of people, and according to my father, you took care of them personally at home. Then, there was Lucille.

LUCILLE—ONE-ROOM SCHOOLS TO ALZHEIMER'S
ADVANCE WORK

As a teacher, Lucille could relate to kids who were fearful and anxious about school. She knew how they felt. She ran away from school on her first day. Granddad took her back. Eventually, though, she started to take to school. She earned an elementary school teaching certificate before she graduated from high school and went on to teacher's college. She taught twenty years in one-room schools with names like Beech Hill, Oak Hill, Gravel Hill, Two Run, and Red Mud. Many were gone when she retired in 1980 and she was teaching in a four-room school in Clover.

By 1970, Lucille started taking care of Grandmother and Granddad, who were just entering their eighties. Lucille's husband, Clark, had died and Lucille was still teaching. "Grandmother's memory" was as close as we came to a diagnosis as I remember it. So, Alzheimer's slipped in unannounced. Granddad had diabetes and heart problems, but his mind was sharp and he could watch Grandmother during the day. And Lucille was there to help with meals and to take laundry to the laundromat eighteen miles away in Spencer.

*

After two years, things changed. Lucille, who had been letting routine screenings like pap smears slide, got caught. Advanced, stage IV cervical cancer. "A fifteen percent likely survival rate for one year," my mother whispered into the phone to me.

Lucille stayed with Uncle Herbert and Aunt Maude in Baltimore and received treatment at Johns Hopkins. I lived near Annapolis then, and on weekends I would spend time with the Baltimore Garretts and Lucille. Lucille was nothing short of stunning in her handling of her cancer and treatment. She would spend a week in isolation getting some kind of implanted radiation and then, next thing you knew, she was sitting around the kitchen table in Baltimore asking for sauerkraut. Her general good health and strength were phenomenal.

Check-ups gave her a clean bill of health until a few years out. Then cancer cells showed up in the lymph glands. More treatment. Success again. Lucille was determined to take care of Grandmother and Granddad, and she did. She cared for them 'til the end with the aid of my mother, who went to help with hands-on care for the last weeks of Granddad and Grandmother's lives, since Lucille was still working. The two sisters made a good team.

While Lucille was doing her caregiving, I wasn't paying that much attention. I was just living my life and working to build a career.

Granddad died in 1977 at the age of eighty-eight. I remember vividly a couple of scenes from Granddad's funeral. First, the room at the funeral home was packed with people, country people who had come to pay tribute to Ed Garrett. He was one of them. Their clothes were work clothes, not fancy suits. They were clean and ever so respectful. Then, as the funeral cortege led out of town to the rural cemetery, I turned to look back. The road curved through a valley. In that one glance I could see cars and trucks, coated with red clay dust and mud with their lights on. The line wrapped from one hill to the next. I was touched.

Grandmother died two years later at the age of ninety. Her demeanor was still kind and gentle, but her mind had given way to Alzheimer's years before. As Lucille had cared for Granddad and Grandmother, she had kept the challenges of her own cancer at bay.

In my own life, I became a US Senate staffer and came to enjoy the stories and work of politics. Technically I was a press aide, speechwriter, and writer of special letters. Sometimes, not often, I did advance work. The advance man or woman tended to every major and minor detail to see that things happened in a way that supported the principal. That's also what family caregivers do.

Caregivers pay bills, make health care appointments, arrange for healthcare providers with specific skills, and decide placement in specialized housing if necessary. Cheerleaders. Fixers. Advocates. Their work, helping to prepare for the end, can go on for years. In politics, advance people are high-energy kids. Grown-ups can't take it for long. In reality, caregivers are the advance staff for those who are dying. Family caregivers are unpaid, but committed to comfort, kindness, and good cheer in the most dire of circumstances. Lucille was an advance person for Granddad and Grandmother. She was my model, though I didn't know it at the time.

Two years after her caregiving was over, Lucille's health failed. She collapsed at home quietly, silently. Daughter Candace broke the door down to get her to the hospital. As the seriousness of her condition became clear, more than a hundred people stopped by the hospital to wish her well. "You won't need an open casket," Lucille announced to her daughters. "All of Roane County has been through here."

Later she returned to Johns Hopkins in Baltimore, where she courageously decided against treatment for this new highly aggressive leukemia. I was there at her insistence when she made the decision, and I was stunned when the "no" came out of her mouth. But, I was her advance person for that part of her journey. It was the most memorable and powerful experience of my life. She was strength and courage personified. Decades later, that experience was the foundation for my commitment to family and my role in end-of-life care. The messages of care and responsibility had become ingrained as a result of my extended family's example.

In her final days in West Virginia, her daughters, Candace and Kate, and my mother were her advance people.

"Your voice sounds frail," I told my mother on the phone in West Virginia.

"Crying," she told me in a matter-of-fact tone. "It's so hard on her."

My mother had parked the car in the hospital lot on Sunday and she hadn't moved it. Candace would relieve her tonight, despite the fact that she would teach school tomorrow.

*

Lucille's advance work for Grandmother and Granddad was over; she could leave now and rest. She died two years after grandmother's death. I didn't know it then, but she fit the pattern for the statistics on caregiving mortality: more than a sixty percent chance of dying within four years after caregiving ends.[10] In addition, my mother lost her best friend of more than sixty-five years. This loss sent her into the darkest grief and years of mourning and depression.

---

10. Schulz and Beach, "Caregiving as a Risk Factor for Mortality," 2215-2219.

Dad's Health Challenges

As 2002 began, Dad's health challenges needed attention. He needed bone surgery around both eyes to make more room for the optic nerve. First one eye, then the other. Both were outpatient surgeries. So, there I was planning to take our Alzheimer's patient along on our little outpatient surgery adventure to Lansing, fifty miles away.

Weather. Aye, snow followed by ice. Cold, nasty, and treacherous. Surgery was re-scheduled. Even though the big storm was over, there were still snow squalls and low visibility. In the waiting room a week later, Mother and I went through every magazine in the place. Dad's surgery seemed longer than we were led to believe it would be. It was later than we expected by the time we got in the car and headed home. After more than thirty years in the South, I had less confidence in my snow and ice driving skills. So, I don't mind telling you my anxiety level was high. Driving a rented car. Both hands on the wheel. As the sun went down, it was harder to tell the lanes. Traffic was heavy until we got about fifteen miles out of Lansing. Check the mirrors. Check the lanes.

Suddenly, there was a heavy, urgent jab on my right arm. I started to turn to say that I needed to keep my eyes on the road. From the back seat, Miss Dixie pointed to the blood streaming down my dad's face. *Geez Louise, now what?* Of course, I had just a couple of tissues in my purse. Minor problem, it turned out. But, I swear that little trip took two years off my life. And Miss Dixie's judgment, despite her Alzheimer's, was on target. She helped take care of Dad on the trip home. All those years together. Still looking after each other no matter what the limitations were. I remembered an earlier time before Alzheimer's when he was hospitalized for gall bladder surgery. It was January and the weather was icy. In the middle of the night, unable to sleep, my mother slid her way on treacherously icy roads to the hospital. She needed to see her husband

and be with him.

Years later, somehow we made it home, got inside the house, and got Dad settled into his chair, which was where he wanted to be. This caring for two people wasn't for sissies. We lived through this surgery and another one in the summer.

*

Again in the spring, I went to Michigan. Mother was still very sweet, but her confusion and agitation were increasing. I had told someone in Virginia that she could still dress herself, although on this trip it seemed more difficult for her than I remembered. However, in spite of this she apologized to a health care worker about the ragged condition of her fingernail polish.

In another conversation, she said, "I'm going to be an idiot." She recognized her impairment on one level, but was unable to do anything about it on another.

One of the most heart-wrenching conversations I had with her was when I was helping her in the shower. She was completely exhausted from the ordeal of washing her hair and showering. Physically shaking she said, "I'm not sure how much longer I want to live."

Her tone was matter-of-fact. It wasn't maudlin or baiting for a response from me. It was said with a gentle disclaimer, which I can no longer remember, that implied she was not going to take any action on it, but that the feeling was there.

The personal hygiene issue became Dad's greatest frustration. She smelled and refused to clean herself up. When I was home, I would help her and try to show her how to do things safely. I was still hoping she would remember. Dumb on my part. She was unwilling to accept Dad's help with the shower, but she would accept mine. Eventually, we wised up and arranged through the county office on aging for a wonderful woman to come in to help weekly with showering and hair washing. Crisis resolved.

To someone looking in on Alzheimer's caregiving, this solution might seem obvious. But, caregiving solutions were much more trial-and-error than obvious. What if the patient fought the solution? When I tried a similar solution in Arlington County, it absolutely did not work. The woman who arrived was poorly trained, failed to connect with mother in any way, and spent the rest of her time in our household yelling at her children on her cell phone in her native language. There were cultural issues in play here, but we couldn't make it work. Even though we were not paying a steep hourly rate, my father, the Scotsman, was outraged. Folks who survived the Great Depression expect value when they spend their hard-earned income and savings. My father was not about to pay for a woman screaming on the phone to her children when she was supposed to be helping my mother.

In between visits to Michigan, I was learning more about Alzheimer's in my support group, from the Internet, and from occasional seminars for caregivers in the DC area. I found myself surprised by all I used from seminars. Suggestions that were almost throwaway lines ended up being as valuable as the main theme. On one occasion, a speaker mentioned casually the use of memory books for Alzheimer's patients in assisted living facilities.

Later, as Mother, Dad, and I were sorting through pictures at the Michigan house, I remembered the memory book idea. Increasingly Mother was asking me about her own history on each visit. "How long have I lived here? How long have I been with him?"

Somehow, I landed on the idea of creating a memory book in PowerPoint. So, the story of Mother's life in a photo book was my Christmas present in 2002.

As a visual communicator, Mother tuned in to the vibrant colors I used. Yes, I ran through a couple of color cartridges, but it was worth it. She could still read, and her association with photos would come back to her as she showed people her life story. It was something she used literally for years. And, I used it when I needed to distract her constructively.

My Dad also liked it. "You can use this at the wake, too," said my father, the thrifty Scotsman. I chose not to dwell on that cheery observation.

In addition, I made a note to myself that I needed to start listing "my learnings" from Mother's Alzheimer moments.

"I'm using the old communications patterns that don't work now," I wrote. "I think explanation will help the communication process, but it doesn't. 'Tomorrow we're going to get a blood test.' I forget she doesn't understand logic and she literally can't remember from one minute to the next.

"Nonetheless, she still recognized when she looks nice. This morning she was very cooperative and delighted with the way she looked. She wanted to show Dad."

But, we had gone through a really rough spot. Both of us lost it.

"She screams at me," she told my dad. And she said of him, "He screams at me and it makes me sick."

I begged her to trust me. I told her I had selected her clothes and would not let her look bad. Eventually she acquiesced, after the angst had gone on for well over an hour.

Afterward, I checked the Alzheimer's Association website for guidance on how I might have handled it differently. To reduce anxiety, it suggested not mentioning the purpose of the clothes search. I told my dad, but I'm not sure he understood completely. He had talked to her for more than fifty years and he was used to his old communication patterns. Dad also had an autocratic manner from time to time that proved to be especially counterproductive. As a kid I used to mutter, "Welcome to Camp Kincaid," under my breath when he was giving orders. With mother, I found myself pausing at least to ask whether I was providing too much information. At different times, I felt guilty about "lying" to Mother. *It took a while, but I got over that!*

By this time, we could use the dining room table for meals and conversations. The shrouded archeological dig had moved on. We were still trying to plan for future care, and our discussion had not been going very well.

*

Cousin Nancy Wood and her husband Gene stopped off for a visit to the folks in Michigan, on their way north. Nancy had called me in Virginia to report the visit. When Dad talked about the Masonic Home, Mother got up and left the room. Nancy and I laughed that there was a message there.

On Mother's Day, Mother was the Energizer bunny. She wore me out with repetitions.

Yet, she was still able to wait reliably in one place in a store, or at least she did on that Saturday, when I went to look for Dad in Home Depot.

She was funny and good-humored. For roughly a year and a half, I had been doing their checks. "I've never heard about that," she said, oblivious to the battle royal eighteen months earlier when I took over the job. But she had no memory of the battle now. One of the blessings of Alzheimer's.

For some reason, it seemed funny to her that I was doing the checks from Virginia. She saw it as a statement of her diminished value to Dad. "Oh, he needs to get him another woman. Just put me out in the yard," she said with gales of laughter and good humor, so much so that I couldn't help but laugh.

Earlier in the day, she had said yes to living with me. Both Mother and Dad had agreed. I couldn't wait to get home to my software program to start drawing an addition that would accommodate Mother and Dad and me, and my little home-based business. Out of the blue, we had a plan for the future. It came from my subconscious as I blurted out: "Come live with me."

HOPE AND A PLAN—2003

Our third year in this journey called Alzheimer's began with our new plan. I would build an addition on my tiny house so that two generations could live together with some level of independence and interdependence. It allowed us to move forward with hope and energy.

The great cleanup was also under way. First, it was the archeological digs of the tables covered with years of unnecessary receipts. Then, we moved extra furniture out of a room that used to be my bedroom and sold a few big pieces, so we could begin to walk through the hallway to the room. When we started, just getting the door open was a big deal. Dad was energetic at this point and he had a project, a big one. Two of the more difficult aspects of the cleanup were the absence of landfills within sixty miles of our house and steep fees for relatively small loads.

In between one of my trips back to Michigan, my old room had been cleared enough so that I could actually use the bed. Dad and the Dream Team. Yahoo! A bed, not the sagging living room sofa for me to sleep on. *Heaven, absolute heaven.*

A spring estate sale or a mini sale was one major cleanup project. We had enough fabric that Mother had bought cheaply to start a yard goods store. A few years earlier, I had made the mistake of telling her about a yard goods sale when I was living in western Pennsylvania and they were visiting. She had nearly filled the van with yard goods that were never used, of course. This lack of judgment was, no doubt, coming from undiagnosed Alzheimer's, but Dad and I couldn't put the riddle together at the time.

We had a ridiculous amount of fabric. An apartment that was attached to the house was vacant, so we were able to set up tables there for a spring mini estate sale. A friend came to Michigan with me to help.

We made a little bit of money, but more importantly we moved a lot of stuff.

Meanwhile, Miss Dixie was staying in the house, mostly watching folks stop and go in to the apartment. She came out once dressed in jeans with a flared skirt over top. Loopy, but not too bad. As we were putting up the signs and balloons to help people find us, she ordered the balloons to be placed higher—and she was absolutely right. Another momentarily lucid evaluation. Loopy one minute, on target the next. Amazing.

In addition to the great cleanup project, I was building the addition to my 900-square-foot house that would accommodate the two generations who were about to start living together.

In my mind, I saw *The Waltons*, the 1970s television show, as the model. The only problem was John Boy had siblings. Lots of them. And in my project, it was just me.

I have always remodeled properties, but I usually had my father to help me think through the purpose and function. His health prohibited that now. I was on my own. This addition was going to take some serious money. Might as well get started on the financial piece.

I applied for a loan. My income alone would not cover the loan I was sure I needed, so my dad and I applied for one together. We got the money in March. Despite the loan, both Dad and I needed to come up with $50,000 apiece in cash for the project. Dad put a mortgage on the house in Michigan and I cashed in my IRAs. My IRAs had taken a hit in one of the market downturns, so re-directing my investment into real estate in the booming Northern Virginia market made some financial sense at the time. That would change, of course.

I got rid of the trees first. That was pricey. A dear friend's husband was an architect, and I started bringing my rinky-dink drawings to meetings with him. He didn't seem too impressed with my software, but I liked it. It allowed me to fit furniture into the rooms and think about what I wanted to bring from Michigan.

The essential elements of the plan were one floor, no steps, doorways wide enough for wheelchairs, and a walk-in shower for my mother's bathroom. My house lot was narrow. We could get wheelchair doorways only on one side. I did all of the meetings with the county planning people so that I could keep costs down and also know what was going on. Trying to move things along, I started shopping the building plans before I had the permits approved.

Of course, despite my religious reading of the procedures online, the permit process hit a snag. Arlington County required a very expensive sounding plan for the Chesapeake Bay Watershed Ordinance. I was nowhere near the Chesapeake Bay, or a body of water for that matter. I was on the middle of a hill. Fortunately for you, the reader, my computer containing the blow-by-blow on this little Chesapeake Bay ordinance adventure crashed. I can hardly remember what the issue was now. But it stopped construction. That I do remember.

As an adult, I've never been adverse to a little over-the-top drama to make a point. Alas, I threw an email hissy fit about the Chesapeake Bay Ordinance. My fit was designed to convince someone in a decision-making capacity that what I wanted to do was sufficiently insignificant when compared to the time and energy it could take to deal with me. Shameful, I know, but it was the only way out that I could think of.

In the meantime, I talked to my family's smartest person, Kincaid Cousin Bob Arnott in Denver, who fortunately was in the business of helping companies comply with environmental regulations. My case, I now argued, could be exempted because no basement was being constructed and no large earthmoving vehicles (just an itty bitty Bobcat) would be used in the project. And I really didn't need a lot of fancy work from an engineer coming up with the kind of detailed earth-placement plan that was implied by the county regulations. I had an architect develop a new drawing, explaining where earth would be moved, and I asked the county to come for a site visit.

In the course of my hissy fit, I had pointed out that poor old innocent me was just trying to put together an addition to my house so I could take care of my dear, sweet, aging, and infirmed parents. Their health was failing quickly and they urgently needed my remedy, which was true. I was pretty sure the county didn't want to see me at a public forum where the media might get a whiff of this. The intent of the regulation was, perhaps, noble in earnestly liberal Arlington County, but frankly I didn't care. It was overkill for my project.

In the meantime, my father was yelling to me over the phone, "I'm gonna be dead before you get that thing built."

Me: "Yeah, well, I know. I'm working on it."

My Childhood Sense of Wellbeing Comes Unglued

In the early 1950s, at a large and fun Kincaid family reunion when I was about eight, my oldest uncle, who was the host, seemed to have a swollen stomach. Actually, more a bloated kind of look. Alarm bells were sounded and my uncle, Hubert, promised to see a doctor. There was one nurse in the family at the time.

Within a few weeks, the report was back and it wasn't good. Polycystic kidneys was his diagnosis—the same disease that had killed my grandfather, according to my nurse aunt.

Life expectancy in the 1950s was, at best, forty-five years. More importantly, polycystic kidneys were hereditary. Once there was one diagnosis, other victims were likely. One aunt, a second aunt, a third aunt... And another uncle who was really a pal died at the age of 30.

Sometime in the late 1960s, early 1970s, one aunt gave her sister a kidney and both lived twenty-plus years. It was one of the early, life-affirming successes in family-member transplants.

For me, I remember the fear created in a ten-year-old at my first family funeral. I had no siblings. My aunts, uncles, and cousins were hundreds of miles away in West Virginia. I was sure I'd be an orphan. That's probably when my fear of being an "only" escalated. A kid with a vivid imagination talking only to herself about a hereditary disease was a dangerous thing. There I was in the outpost of Michigan, away from family. Who would take care of me and on and on? What would happen to me? I remember seeing my father cry for the first time. I was stunned and a little confused. Did men cry? For some reason, I didn't think they did. But back to the more important issue: who would take care of me?

The kidney disease seemed bigger and more important to me than it was or should have been. Despite the science that cleared my risk, it popped up in my mind frequently. For me, polycystic kidneys were the clouds that stifled full-blown joy. In 2012, my cousin, David, was the first of my generation to die from the disease. After two transplants and years of keeping his circumstance at bay, he decided that a life consumed by illness, tests, and probes was no longer worth it. He entered hospice and chose to die. Antibiotics for his most recent life-threatening infection were withdrawn, along with the anti-rejection drugs that kept him alive, but which probably also compromised his autoimmune system. After years of courageously fighting to live, it was time for a different decision.

David's first transplant was in 1987. In 1999, he needed another kidney. By that time, anti-rejection drugs made it possible for the kidney to come from a non-family member, and his wife Monna gave him a kidney.

Once Monna was asked about her gift to David. Her explanation: "He's had my heart since I was nine—why wouldn't I give him a kidney?"

And, as she noted at his funeral, she had twenty-four more years than she was supposed to have. How could she be anything but grateful?

There at the funeral, I sat with another cousin that I had not seen in more than fifteen years. When I shook his hand, it was cold. The cold jolted my memory; he, too, had the disease, and so did his beautiful daughter.

I was spared, however. How can I be anything but grateful! Still, it was always there in my head. Totally and completely irrational, but that was me. What if? Should I have children? *Not a problem, dummy.* Yet, I always wondered.

The kidney disease seemed particularly unfair to the Kincaids, a family that had been steeped in sorrow in its early years. My Kincaid grandfather died when my dad was fourteen in 1930, just as the Depression was emerging. Dad was the eldest of the seven children living at home. His mother, at one point, was forced to consider sending her children to an orphanage. My dad told stories of working as a day laborer on the pipeline for pennies so he could take the money home to his mother.

The Kincaids had a garden, but not a farm like the Garretts. So despite my mother's memories of deprivation in Depression, it's my guess that circumstances were even more dire for the Kincaids. Seven years later my grandmother Florence died at the age of forty-seven, leaving three children under the age of twelve. The orphans, as they described themselves, were taken care of by older siblings and other family members. The two youngest carried a special bond into adulthood as they raised their own families. In addition, their charity and kindness to individuals who needed help was done quietly, but with a seriously compassionate purpose. They understood the pain of homelessness and abandonment, even if death was the cause.

*

For my father, my mother's family was a point of stability and welcome, despite a drinking problem here and there and occasional periods of incarceration (not directly related to drinking). Yes, it was a robustly colorful family with streaks of dysfunction. When my dad asked Granddad Garrett for permission to marry Dixie, Granddad had one question: "You a Democrat?" My dad apparently said he COULD be. So, he went against the grain of his Republican family, but that was kind of a secret.

THE KINCAIDS OF ST. LOUIS, MICHIGAN

Mother and Dad stayed with the dry cleaners for roughly twenty years. Eventually they closed it and lived very modestly on income from rental units and selling cleaning products. And, my dad started working for a plumbing business. There was never much money, but enough to live comfortably. They saw themselves as frugal, hard-working survivors of the Great Depression and World War II. Still, they really weren't equipped financially for their long lives, and especially not for a debilitating illness like Alzheimer's.

When it came time for me to go to college, I was on my own. I stayed out of school for a year, which resulted in the loss of a small scholarship. During that period of time, I was state leader of a youth organization. I traveled more than 20,000 miles through the upper and lower peninsulas of Michigan, and my mother was usually in the car with me, including grueling return trips at two and three in the morning. She was both cheerleader and critic. Not quite a Tiger Mother, but she could have held her own on a reality TV show. I worked part-time at a local newspaper.

When I did go to college, I tried being a regular student in the dorm, but I needed a job and the structure it provided. Not to mention the money.

This is really nutty, I know, but I picked my college based on its football record. Not like I was about to get a football scholarship, but I was so sick of my high school not winning a single solitary football game for all four years while I was in school that I really wanted to see some good football. *I know, I know.*

There was a football gene that dominated in my father's family, and I got it to the point of stupidity. My dad, who played college football, loved my reasoning because that meant he could see some excellent games.

So, off I went to Michigan State University (MSU), a Big Ten powerhouse at the time. I could have gone to the University of Michigan. I had the grades; I was salutatorian. But, poor old Michigan just didn't seem to have the football chops then.

A secondary factor to selecting MSU was that I had met a lot of faculty members in the journalism school through summer workshops, and the college was active in recruiting folks from my area. So, I really liked the professors and the program, but as my dad knew my real reason was football and MSU's national standing.

You know what? It paid off. MSU was Number One in the country. Okay, make that tied for Number One with Notre Dame. (I dispute MSU's Number Two ranking.) And, I was witness to the biggest college football game of the decade. By the way, Wikipedia calls the 1966 game "The Game of the Century." Might be pushing it, but it was big.

My suitemate was Bubba Smith's sister. I'll never forget screaming, "Kill Bubba Kill," from my seat on the sidelines. (I took it personally when Bubba died a couple of years ago.) Then Notre Dame played for a tie. A tie was all they needed to win Number One in the national rankings and that was that. Michigan State was Number Two.

Four, almost five decades later, I continued to cheer against Notre Dame every Saturday that I had the opportunity. Of course, Notre Dame remained the only school in the country that had all its games televised, no matter how bad they were. Well-placed alumni in NBC Sports programming solved that mystery.

East Lansing, Michigan, was wild during the week before the game. Alumni boosters managed to get up in arms because MSU's star defensive player was supposedly harassed by local police. In fact, a car owned by one Charles A. Smith was towed because of unpaid parking tickets. The East Lansing Chief of Police responded, "How was I supposed to know Charles A. Smith was Bubba Smith?" I don't remember the outcome and that's probably just as well.

By that time, I had been working at a local weekly newspaper a couple of years. I had started part-time the first week it was published, and such papers were trending then in affluent suburban communities. Working at the *Towne Courier*, which no longer exists, was a good decision. I worked off and on for a couple of years, left to work as a production assistant for a TV cooking show, and returned later to become managing editor of the paper. It was great writing and editing experience, and I learned a little about layout for offset printing, which was the new technology then.

As a result of my newspaper work, several of my introductory journalism classes were waived. I was able to take a range of other classes that interested me, like political science. Being a traditional college student just didn't work for me. I eventually worked fulltime and went to school part-time. It took me seven years to graduate. This was before student loans and college debt. One of the journalism school professors used to call me the "oldest living senior."

She also provided good mentoring advice. "Always keep a go-to-hell fund," she said. That way if you really feel you have to leave a job, you can. I lost touch with her after several moves. She died of Alzheimer's and her former students had served as guardians and conservators, I learned years later from an obituary.

*

In later years as Alzheimer's took hold, my mother's personality quirks would be forgotten, and, at least to some extent, forgiven. However, there was one thing I really never forgave. When I was in college, I used to work hard trying to make tuition, which was an enormous $100 per term. Rent and food were extra, of course. Fortunately, I loved tuna fish and it was about thirty-three cents for a six-ounce can then. I actually made it through one whole week with $1 to my name.

So what did my mother do? Without a word to me, she cashed my income tax refund that, yes, I was counting on for summer tuition. What did she do with it? Bought a piece of furniture. An antique walnut hall tree. A freakin' piece of non-essential furniture. There it stood by the front door: at least seven feet tall, a mirror, an umbrella stand that was never used, and hooks for coats that were never used. My summer tuition stood in the hall by the door for forty-plus years. I kicked it a couple of times.

Fury. Outrage. Dixie didn't seem to notice that my hair was on fire because I was so angry. That was when I stopped going home. I suspect I said something, but I don't remember what it might have been. She had crossed the line.

From then on, all mail, including tax refunds, came directly to me in East Lansing/Okemos. She would ask me for loans through the years and I would give her the money when I had it. But, I carried that old bitterness over that stupid piece of furniture much too long. Forty years later that miserable hall tree brought only $800 in the estate sale. Maybe it was damaged by my kicks and bumps. Funny thing was, I probably would have liked the way the furniture piece looked if I had not hated the way it was acquired. Never would I have liked it well enough to own it, though.

In the last year that my dad was alive, I finally told him the story.

"I never knew about it," he said, and I was sure that was true. "I wondered why you didn't come home anymore." My mother could be astonishingly self-absorbed. A total blind spot. She could also be generous and giving. It was sometimes hard to figure out which Dixie was showing up that day.

My cousins, Kate and Candace, did not see my mother as a self-absorbed person. When Granddad was dying, mother came in almost like a hospice worker for three of four weeks giving care in those last days. The same with Grandmother and her sister Lucille.

In the early days, she could blow into rural West Virginia with a project list, like new siding for the little homestead house, and all farm work stopped until the project was completed. It was an all-hands-on-deck project. Uncle Russell, who farmed the homestead, stopped farming and picked up a hammer along with my dad, who worked nonstop. Someone once asked me how she could get people to cooperate, and I never had a good answer for that. You simply didn't argue with the logic of the Tiger Project person. "No," was an unacceptable response, and there would be hell to pay. She knew how to set a fire under people and she wasn't afraid to do it.

"Yes, I could call her a pain," my cousin Kate said, "but in truth we needed that sometimes." And, they remember her generosity and thoughtfulness, which is a wonderful thing.

Her end-of-life care for family members was very important to her, and Dixie was understandably proud of being there and caring. I think she viewed her presence during those times as her ultimate statement of love. She often said it was the most important thing she had done in her life. There was that side of her, but there was another side that I saw. I couldn't tell which Dixie was going to show up—the kind and generous person or the self-absorbed person. Her judgmental kid was watching all the moves and quarterbacking the motivation game on Monday morning.

*

Sometime after the Alzheimer's diagnosis, Dad and I were sitting in the family room talking about living options. I was reminded of the social worker at the medical practice in Lansing who said to him, "This is a lot for you to take on. How do you feel about it?"

"Not bad," he said. "It could have been the other way around and she could be taking care of me." They had been married 61 years. Perhaps the pain of his family's early years made it easier for him to accept his new role of caregiver. He had learned early that life could be unfair. Had it not been for my dad, my life would have been hell. No doubt about it.

I don't quite know how to explain this, but my mother's coping skills were pretty limited.

On the plus side, she let me do lots of things that other mothers might not. When I was four, I made a cake. *Well, kind of. I think the truth was I stirred a cake and helped pour it into a cake pan.*

But my favorite story was another cooking exercise. I was about ten and empowered to operate heavy equipment—the mixer, the stove, the oven, probably the old wringer washing machine, certainly the vacuum cleaner. I wasn't terribly impressed with the fact I was authorized to use this stuff, since it seemed pretty clear to me that my mother's motivation was self-serving.

"Barbara, run the vacuum. Cook lunch or supper." True, she worked in the dry cleaners and it was physically demanding. But...

There I was, probably making a cake with the mixer. It was a weekend, since Mother was sitting at the kitchen table. Anyway, I said something profound and descriptive like, "Oops. Got my hand caught." Next thing I knew, she was doing a drama queen number.

"Oh my goodness, you'll be ruined. I'm going to be sick. What should I do?"

"Well," said I. "Could you maybe pull the plug! So the mixer turns off?"

"Oh," she said. I looked at her and thought, *what a screw-up,* and went on to finish the mixer project, whatever it was.

"She was a good mother," my dad said. Now, as I think back, I note that he didn't say she was a good wife. Should I have registered that question while he was alive? Since I never really shared his assessment of her mothering skills, I probably tried to change the subject. She certainly wasn't bad, but "good?" My list of grievances was substantial. First, she became a victim and dependent personality very quickly. She didn't know the first thing about taking care of herself.

I've never forgotten the time she called me at my eighty-hour-a-week job. My dad was working out of town. Mother demanded that I drive forty miles to meet her and give her my house key because she had locked herself out. By this time, I was living in an apartment and had enough sense to hide a key somewhere. Why couldn't she? She was a screw-up.

Then, there was the boss at my newspaper job, and yes—I was going to school, too. My mother, the omnipotent pain in the ass, had called my boss to tell him he was working me too hard. The woman was unbelievable.

Later, when I had major surgery, I didn't tell her until it was over because I didn't want her anywhere near me. Why? I would have to take care of HER. So, I went to my aunt and uncle's house the first time, and the second time I went home by myself. And I kept my plans a secret until the surgery was over.

I used to think that the most important part of the gift of my mother having Alzheimer's was that I had to forget and forgive some of those old bitter incidents. So much of family relationships was based on shared memories; some good, some not. Then the memory was gone. The glue and bond was weakened. But so was the bitterness. Few, or more probably no family relationships are perfect. Still, I never believed that imperfection should spare me the responsibility to care for my parents. If not me, who? I also discovered that spouses, friends, and family who can focus on the present, not future expectations or the past, are the most comfortable with caregiving. It's an adjustment, but one I found less difficult than I first believed it would be.

In the early stage when she came to visit, she wouldn't stop talking. She would sit on my bed and I would end up begging her to let me go to sleep, since I needed to go to work the next day.

Mother loved the telephone, and the phone was our primary communication tool. Face-time visits were usually limited to once, maybe twice a year. There were exceptions when something of interest happened in the DC area. When the Impressionist exhibit was featured at the National Gallery of Art, my parents came to visit because my mother had started painting when she was sixty. Both Dad and I were really proud of Mother's paintings. Like sewing and cooking, she was really focused on learning how to do it well. She took classes with the Art Guild and read books on technique. But, the books and the paintings at the National Gallery from the Impressionist exhibit were special. We went three different times for HOURS. She would study the light, composition, and brushstrokes of each painting and come home, read the catalog and books from the bookshop, then return again. Although I was starting to tire of going there, she would literally start to cry to be taken back again. *Okay, okay.* So of course, I took her again.

Even now as I look at her paintings, I am awed by her talent. The clouds she painted are special and nuanced. There is energy in the sky above trees and barns. I was not sure, but always believed she got interested in paintings watching public television. Her use of color is lovely. Still life subjects were her focus, though one of her first paintings was of the sweet dog that lived next door. Barns and scenes from her childhood were favorites, along with flowers from her yard in interesting, occasionally antique containers.

Right after college graduation, I was hired by the late Philip A Hart, a Democratic United States Senator from Michigan. What got me the job was my ability to do layout for offset printing. It was good that I could write, but not essential. Another positive factor was my experience with weekly newspapers. At that point I had worked for two weekly newspapers. Weeklies were big outside of the state's metropolitan areas, and Michigan was a big state with lots of rural counties.

By far the most important element of my job was to produce letters of condolence for casualties of the Vietnam War from Michigan. Each of these notes was personally signed by the senator; no automated pen signer was ever used. It was easy and depressing to chart the course of the Vietnam War by the casualty list. So, my life on the East Coast in metropolitan Washington, DC, began while my parents continued to live in rural central Michigan.

One Step Forward At Last

At long last, the Arlington house addition seemed ready to move ahead. The county zoning staff needed to visit the construction site to see if the case I had outlined about the Chesapeake Bay Ordinance was viable. It was, and I nearly did a handstand. Speeding out of my driveway, I almost ran over the nice man who gave me the approval. Get that permit before the county office closed. The nice man smiled, maybe laughed. Construction started the next day, a Saturday.

We began late. One of the first problems occurred quickly. The original house was six inches closer to a side property line than it should have been. The architect's drawing set the side of the addition into the required county side-yard distance. The contractor missed it; I didn't and the foundation was re-done.

Back in Michigan, Mother's disease was progressing. Not rapidly, but progressing. Dad's thyroid was eliminated by a radioactive medication and he was waiting to see if more was needed. His energy level was low. Mother was having trouble understanding that I couldn't stay with her because I needed to get back to work. She said she was afraid to go to sleep and that she was afraid of the dark.

Nonetheless, one early morning about six, I was aroused from my sleep by the sound of happy feet coming down the hallway. My door creaked open and a sweet-sounding voice said, "Hi, it's me. Are you awake? It's me."

"Go back to bed," I growled, and turned over. Back the happy feet went.

There were other, more difficult moments. One of my birthdays began at five in the morning with Mother distressed because she had wet the bed. She was not yet using adult diapers, and I had just put a mattress cover with a plastic liner on her side of the bed. As her disease advanced, getting her corralled when she had diarrhea became difficult. It was as though she recognized it as loss of control and believed if she ran from it that would fix the situation. Not to be too graphic, but her trail made life more difficult than it needed to be.

That particular morning we just changed her clothes. "You know, I don't know how much longer I want to live like this," she said. Most of the time there were no expressions of sadness from her, but for some reason this day was different. She fell right back to sleep, but I couldn't. I cried. *Happy Birthday to me.* Then, I yelled at myself. *Suck it up, wimp.*

One of the challenges to staying in step with the "best practices" for Alzheimer's care was tuning in to international advances. More seemed to happen internationally than it did in the US, particularly with medications. For example, the drug memantine had been used in Germany since 1982, and by 2003 it was available in 42 countries outside the United States.[11] Despite the fact that it was first produced in the US, it was not available for US patients. A number of Alzheimer's advocates saw this as unreasonable. Yes, the data were mixed on its efficacy as a mid-stage medication. But let's get real, the advocates said, there was nothing else out there, except versions of one other basic medication. Something that MIGHT help was better than nothing. So, the Food and Drug Administration (FDA), after hearings, let the medication go on the market in the US.

The history of this medication illustrated how hard it was to stay abreast of what might be done and advocate for investment in research, or the fast tracking of medications—as was done with AIDS and HIV. Why do you suppose that was? One of my theories started with the fact that Alzheimer's was an old person's disease. AIDS and HIV often took people in their most productive years. We as a society were stunned by the loss of talent and skill in the AIDS epidemic. Not so with Alzheimer's, at least on the face of it. These kinds of assumptions, of course, were shallow and ignored the impact of Alzheimer's during the productive years of family caregivers, not to mention early onset Alzheimer's.

The Alzheimer's I came to know crossed generations. I had every intention of working until I was seventy and beyond. As the physical

11. Forest Labs, Inc., "Memantine HCl," 13, August 20, 2003, http://www.fda.gov/ohrms/dockets/ac/03/briefing/3979B1_01_ForestLabs-Memantine.pdf.

challenges to caregiving increased, my own health began to fail and I was forced to retire early. In the early years, of course, I had no idea that would happen.

Besides, as a hands-on caregiver, I had too much to do to try to plot rocking the boat as an Alzheimer's advocate. I certainly didn't have time to snarl at whomever or whatever about shortcomings in attention to Alzheimer's as a policy and research issue. There I was, working, trying to earn a living to pay for a new mortgage, overseeing a building project, and traveling back and forth to Michigan every six weeks to help my father. *A full life...* Analyzing the research shortcomings and advocating a change in priorities was pretty far down on my to-do list.

However, during my occasional down time, I gave some thought to how I needed to frame the work—caregiving—that I was beginning. Alzheimer's is terminal. There is no cure, no way to prevent it. Roughly five million have the disease in the US. More than fifteen million are family caregivers.[12]

I tended to think of issues as win/lose. I was going to invest emotionally in a significant way and I would fail. No matter how hard I tried, my mother would die. Maybe my dad would survive longer, but not my mother. So my objectives and purposes needed a different framework. I began to try to redefine success as bringing as much joy and comfort to Mother and Dad in their later years as possible. Happiness, joy, and comfort were the metrics of my new definition of success.

That definition became an important step in helping me understand the limitations of my effort on outcomes. Of course, much of the problem was that I had bought into a traditional, largely romantic concept of success, also known as the American dream. You know: the win/lose/climb thing. I was a non-traditional practitioner of the American dream for females. I wasn't a boomer, I was a member of the Silent Generation. I was unmarried and childless. I was not destined to be President of the United States or president of anything else, for that matter. *So what. Not a big deal.*

When people referred to ALL I was giving up to take care of my parents, it was difficult not to laugh. My career was humorous; it lacked focus and commitment. For the last twenty years, I had not taken my

---

12. Alzheimer's Association, "2011 Alzheimer's Disease Facts and Figures," http://www.alz.org/downloads/facts_figures_2011.pdf.

career very seriously. Indeed, I concluded that I had probably made a serious error in judgment by believing that a career was what I'd wanted in the first place. At that point, I had had jobs, but a career? I had changed professional directions a couple of times. Was I a failure, then? Perhaps, but oddly I was and am reluctant to say that. Failure seemed a little severe, since I really liked what I did. I had had a lot of fun. Sure, there were jobs that I'd hated, but I had found jobs that I loved. Still, it was not like I was on the brink of finding a cure for cancer or Alzheimer's. That's what I would call a career worthy of commitment. Mine? Not so much. So what was I giving up?

The other side of the issue was that I really enjoyed working. As a partner in a consulting firm, I could be selective about individual clients and cautious about matching personalities and operating styles. I figured I would work at least part time until my late seventies. Little did I know.

LATE AT NIGHT: TIME FOR REFLECTION

I could think, write, read, or meditate late at night. Sometimes my time was spent on work; sometimes it was spent remembering the good decisions I'd made. Or the bad. Sometimes it was spent in silence with the mind slowed. How hard one has to work to be mindless—or mind*ful*, as the state is so often described these days!

Sitting at the computer years later in Arlington, I would sometimes glance at the bookshelf above. A handwritten letter was framed on paper, now yellowed, which served as a reminder of how long ago it was. The date says 8/23/1974 and it is on Philip A. Hart's small letterhead. The handwriting was Senator Hart's familiar scrawl.

"Barb," he started out. *I hate being called Barb; I prefer Barbara. Barb is kind of a Michigan thing. The minute you cross the state line, you will be known as BARB. Was I going to tell a US Senator not to call me Barb? No.* The senator continued:

"Please do a note to Barbara K. Kincaid. (Florence has address) (Believe not married)

"Understand she has had a difficult time lately (physical, not mental). Hope she is feeling much better.

"If anything office or I can do, pls [sic] let us know.

"Janey would join me etc. but haven't seen her since 4th of July weekend in St. Thomas.

"Explain delay in writing (a) compelling national events (b) absence of my writer (c)... you can handle it I know.

"Indicate very real hope that she will be fully active soon; that she has been missed by all of us!

"Thanks—

"Sign it 'Phil Hart.' "

*

So in this typically wry, cryptic piece of inside humor, Philip A. Hart (or PAH, as we called him) was telling me to do a note to myself. Some further decoding is in order here: "compelling national events" referred to President Nixon's resignation, and "absence of my writer" was *MY* absence. Since no one confessed to putting him up to this, I think it really did come from him. Sometimes I would type things out for him and suggest that he handwrite it, but no one came forward on this one so it's likely from him.

Every now and then, PAH would stick his head in the office to tell me he was going to need some jokes for a weekend speech. That always annoyed Jack Cornman, the chief speechwriter during this period. "He didn't ask *me* for jokes," Jack would pout. *No, Jack, you don't write funny.* Instead, he was the memorable rhetoric guy. His stuff was etched in stone. Stone versus jokes; I think that evens out.

Sometimes, I would wonder how different my life would have been if I hadn't taken the Senate job. I had done one interview with Gannett in East Lansing and was scheduled for a trip to Rochester, New York, for a second interview. The Gannett recruiter was a high-level former executive. When I wrote to tell him of my change in plans he minced no words about the mistake I was making. He took my decision very personally and had talked to me about a long-term career with Gannett. I always wondered what if...

Learning from my First Friend in DC

My first friend in DC was Martha. We were about the same age, late twenties, working together in the same Senate office. She was shorter than I was, very petite, and had great, shiny, dark brown hair. She was from Michigan by way of Haight-Ashbury in San Francisco. I was in my blonde phase, which lasted about twenty years. And, yes, blondes do have more fun, assuming their hair doesn't fall out from too many chemicals.

How long was Martha in the hippie land of Haight-Ashbury? Seemed like a year or so until she settled down and literally got off the drug-induced high. I was such a goodie-goodie by comparison. By the time I knew her, smoking cigarettes and drinking were our shared vices, often on the floor of her apartment or mine. We lived one whole block from each other; neither had a car. I lived about a block and a half from the office. Martha was closer.

Our conversations usually focused on books, music, and men. And office gossip, of course. Martha was on the front line at the reception desk answering the phone during the Vietnam protest days. I was hidden away back in the press office. During a full moon, when they needed to get a telephone conversation away from the reception desk, the press office would sometimes get the overflow. But that didn't happen often.

Washington and Capitol Hill, in particular, were tough crime spots then. Martha was always getting mugged, grabbed from behind and robbed of her purse, but nothing really bad happened to me. Actually I should revise that a bit. The cousin of my boyfriend was shot and died in a typical-for-the-time mugging that went badly. The cousin was a law student and I had just met him briefly. But that's another story.

*

Martha liked to walk after work to the grocery store, which was maybe five blocks away. That was customarily when she got mugged. I was a sissy. I didn't like that store anyway. So, I stayed inside after dark, which started at 4 o'clock in the winter. I remember my mother being outraged that I had to work at night. I laughed at her. In retrospect, I was lucky she didn't call Senator Hart as she did an earlier boss to tell him he should let me leave work while it was light out. Trust me, that call never would have gotten through.

Both Martha and I had long-distance men in our lives. Mine was in upstate New York; hers was in Michigan. I think hers might have been married and a former Congressman. Mine was very single and a boyfriend from college. Things got very secretive when her boyfriend came to town. We both had trouble fitting in and belonging in Washington.

She gave up on DC before I did and went to work in our Detroit office while she finished her degree. She had a wonderful apartment in Birmingham, and I stayed there once on my way to central Michigan. She had just a couple more classes before she was through with school. Martha was exceedingly bright and gave some consideration to getting a PhD. in literature. We would touch base frequently on the office phone. I was getting happier with my life in Washington, although technically it was outside DC. And I was getting more connected with people in the region.

One Friday afternoon in March we had a long conversation on the phone. Then two, maybe three days, later, Martha was dead.

Suicide.

She had put her favorite classical music album on the stereo, put on her best dress, and hanged herself with a bicycle chain. Her sister, Sylvia—whom she loved dearly—found her. I was a basket case. The senator went back for the funeral. The office offered to send me because we were known to be close friends, but I just couldn't do it. I couldn't face it. By that time I had given up on living in the city and had moved to a little waterfront house, near the Chesapeake Bay. I took the day off and sat on the end of my dock in Cypress Creek, talking to the ducks. Asking, "Why?"

I carried guilt for not "getting it" for weeks, months. At some point, I added anger to the brew. Why didn't she tell anyone? Anger at what she did to her sister. On and on. Meaning I really didn't get it. It stayed with me, too. Off and on for years. Why? How could she do that to her sister?

As stunning and important as this was to me, I don't remember how I heard of her death. But I remember the timeframe: the Ides of March.

*

A few years later, I hit a level of despondency that helped me understand. I didn't have the motivation to act, but I came to a better understanding of her despair and the absence of hope. I came through it and was grateful for what despair taught me. This may sound very odd, but sometimes I see suicide as a very rational choice. When I read in the press of a suicide pact between a husband and wife after one has an Alzheimer's diagnosis, I get it and honor their choice. Or at least I think I do.

*

For a while it seemed to me as though death was stalking my friends. Both college roommates lost their last parent. Such an odd coincidence. I fretted about what the universe was telling me in those situations. Add to that President Kennedy's assassination when I was in school, and grief was beginning to become part of my curriculum. I had a genuinely prophetic moment a couple of weeks before the President's death when I told a roommate, as we were changing bed linens, that I had a feeling something really awful was about to happen. Worse than we could even imagine. When November 22, 1963, happened, both of us remembered the conversation.

The President's death was also the first time I discovered that the headache I got at funerals didn't come from a flower allergy. I had my customary funeral headache at Kennedy's funeral as we all watched in the dorm lounge, but there were no flowers. Loss and grief had physical symptoms, I learned by the time I finished college. Martin Luther King and Robert Kennedy died just before I finished working my way through school. My melancholy and association with the dark side of life was accelerating. "The black hole," I have frequently called it. I had trouble shaking it. Was it because I was a journalism student and I really focused on national events and commentary? Or, was it because as a kid I had obsessed so much over the early deaths in my dad's family? I still remember a television discussion (in black and white, of course) with the Rev. William Sloane Coffin Jr., a noted minister from Yale and later the influential Riverside Church in New York. He said something like the most important and powerful connection between people, even those who disagree, is "how much have you suffered?" He meant real loss, death, and bereavement. It implied that an openness to sharing suffering could lead to a connection that was particularly strong. It stayed with me through the years.

*

Years later, I stood in my kitchen in a house I was renting in a Philadelphia suburb and was stunned by a casual statement from my friend's husband. The subject was Alzheimer's. His father had died of Alzheimer's before any medications were available and the experience had been brutal, including flawed business decisions made when no one knew he had the disease. Here was a case of a bright, politically connected man brought down by Alzheimer's before anyone understood what might be happening.

"I'm not putting *my* family through it," he said. "I'll commit suicide first." I turned to look at him and felt a deep chill as I looked in his eyes. He meant it. A year or so later he took his own life. Still, I was stunned and incredulous. "He thought he was getting Alzheimer's," my friend reported after the fact, as she recalled a startling incident when her husband was lost on the subway and couldn't even remember the purpose of his trip.

Once again, I was angry at what he did to his daughter and wife.

Later I would have my own despair and would finally reach a level of empathy and forgiveness. It seemed that I needed to experience my own deep despair before I could really accept his—and Martha's, for that matter. It is still shocking to me how long that process can take. Honoring choices and decisions must be the grace of wisdom. I hope someday to reach its presence quickly and without anger. A sensitivity to the pain, yes, but not anger.

A Frightening Interlude

In Michigan at Christmas 2003, Doc Hall reported a new concern with my father's health. Keeping his blood count at a healthy level was increasingly a challenge, he said. In truth, I had so much going on—building an addition, running my business from home, and long-distance family caregiving—that the significance of this new wrinkle didn't register as much as it probably should have.

The folks would move to Virginia by June of 2004. That's what I was saying, but I was hoping we could get it accomplished sooner. The builder fortunately was focused on my project and my project alone. So we were spared the usual problems with sub-contractors. There were some scheduling problems, but not the nightmare stories that you so often hear about.

The roof was on, the block and stucco for the exterior walls were finished, the windows were in. The interior walls were being roughed in. The electrical work was moving along.

*

January 22, 2004. My telephone rang about 10 a.m. Caller ID told me it was my dad calling at an unusual time of day.

"Well, how are you?" I said cheerfully.

"Had a terrible night. Couldn't reach any of those numbers," he said, meaning the numbers I had put in large print. His vision, though improved, was still a problem. Shocked, I shifted gears quickly. He happened to hit my phone number because I had programmed it into his phone. His voice was frail and halting.

Clearly, he was a very sick man. Did he say he was lying on the floor in the bedroom maybe all night? I think he did.

I told him I'd get right on it. Help was on the way. I would get on the phone.

I called neighbor Dave Zimmerman and left word. Dr. Hall's office, then his home. He wasn't there but his wife, Ann, answered. Doc was in the Emergency Room (ER) and she would call him to let him know that Dad was on his way in. I would never have been able to get through to him as quickly as she did.

Grant Colthorp, who had Dad's medical power of attorney, was next. He had a house key and would get Dad to the ER as fast as he could. The odd thing was I didn't really think about Mother, who could no longer be left alone. She was forgotten temporarily in this new crisis.

Then I started looking for flights to get me to central Michigan as fast as possible. I found one leaving from Baltimore Washington International (BWI) to Lansing. The next thing was to get a ride to BWI. I started calling people: a former boyfriend, my friend Lynne. Meanwhile, the electrician was scheduled to start doing the electrical work and I absolutely had to spot all of the lights for the addition construction. Who knew how long I might be gone?

Sometime later after Dad was in the hospital, I called the house. I had lost track of time. Mother answered the phone.

"Are you by yourself?" I asked.

"Oh no," she said. "What's your name?"

"Ann Hall," a voice close by said. In the absence of other options, Doc Hall's wife Ann had come to stay with my mother. Amazing, truly amazing... the kindness and commitment of the Barbershoppers' Fab Four. Would I ever be able to sufficiently express my gratitude?

"Dad went to the hospital," I said to Mother, checking to see if she understood. "Yes, I'm glad you called," she said very simply. "I'll be home tomorrow," I told her.

Later Dave Zimmerman had called, I learned after the fact. Mother answered.

"Who's with you?" Dave asked. "A friend," Mother reported. "Who's the friend?" Mother said she didn't know.

"May I talk with her?" Dave asked.

"No," said Mother. "You don't know her." Click! And she hung up the phone.

That evening Doc Hall called to report on Dad's condition and to tell me I needed to get to Michigan soon. He was guarded about any prognosis other than "not good." Double bacterial pneumonia along with anemia. The anemia diagnosis would change to myelodysplastic syndrome, which the National Institute of Health (NIH) website called smoldering leukemia.

Overnight in Arlington... freezing rain on top of a base of light snow. At 6:30 the next morning, I did a walk-through with the contractor on the electrical work. Light here, switch here, here. In my rush, the only significant mistake I made was placing the lights I wanted over the dining room table. I ended up using the table in a different configuration, and every time I looked up at the ceiling my error in judgment annoyed me. But at the time, it was more important to get to Michigan while my father was still alive.

I walked gingerly down the driveway to Lynne's car. Such an odd confluence of sorrow yet solidarity. Lynne would turn west from BWI and head to Frostburg to be with her mother in her final hours. We had been friends supporting each other through multiple sorrows for more than thirty years, including the death of her first husband from a self-inflicted gunshot.

On Friday at 12:40 p.m. I looked at my watch and was overwhelmed with sadness and sorrow. I was in a small propjet in the snow-filled skies between Cleveland and Lansing. We were flying low enough so that I could see the patterns of the farmland below. It was a distinctive moment, and I was so afraid it was a premonition of my father dying. In retrospect, it may have been empathy for Lynne. She arrived at noon and her mother died at 1:15 p.m.

I arrived at home in St. Louis to find neighbor Deb Zimmerman with my mother. My father had been stabilized and was in isolation. Grant had arranged for a caregiver to stay overnight in the house with mother. All I had to do was pay her. Friends and neighbors were trading off on daytime hours until I could get there. I kept saying over and over to myself, *"Thank you. He's alive."*

Beginning the next day, Mother and I were able to spend some brief time with Dad each day. Dad's doctor asked his other friends not to come to the hospital, fearful that he might get something else. He cried when he saw Mother come through the hospital room door in a wheelchair, all dolled up with a mask, gloves, and clothing covers. Getting ready to go, she put makeup on independently and asked me to find her nail polish; then she put it on herself.

Dad was very emotional, since he'd thought Wednesday night and Thursday morning that he was going to die. By the weekend, he was saying, "You know, I think I can come out of this." He started lobbying to come home.

When we were back at the house, Mother would realize Dad was gone and sometimes remembered where he was. Then, she would say she was anxious to see him. Can we go now to see him? Why can't we go now?

There at the hospital, she told him: "I think you're better. Your eyes are brighter."

And he said: "I think I feel a little better." *Ah yes, the will to live.*

*

In Denver, another family sorrow was playing out. Kincaid Cousin Bob Arnott lost his father, Roma T, at the age of ninety-five. I spoke with Bob and he asked me to tell my dad. I decided to wait a day or two. Roma had married Dad's sister and I was sure my dad would feel the loss tremendously. As Kincaid cousins, Bob and I had been close. Proximity in age meant we often played together at family reunions, and that bond seemed to hold as we got older. Dad and Roma were good friends, talking on the phone often after my aunt's death.

I remembered a favorite scene from Uncle Hobe's. I had heard a conversation floating up in the morning hours and looked out the upstairs window to see three eighty-year-old men below in deep discussion about some pipe down near the kitchen. My dad seemed to be giving a plumbing seminar to Hobe and Roma T. Of the group, my father was youngest. It was a scene of earnest intention and curiosity among the octogenarians. I smiled at the memory of engagement, undiminished by age.

*

What I had forgotten to do in getting Mother ready for her visit with Dad was sanitize the hospital wheelchair, so she came down with a cold on the weekend. Still, we were able to get Dad home and settled in his chair as my week in Michigan was drawing to a close. Should I stay or leave?

We decided it was okay for me to get back to my work and pull some loose ends together. Earlier I had scheduled a trip to Michigan just a week away as a part of my routine every-six-weeks schedule. So the Fab Four could check in on Mother and Dad until I returned.

Besides, I had started planning on an April, not a June move to Virginia for Mother and Dad. Before I left Michigan I told Dad that if it became necessary because of his health to move the transition up even more, all he had to do was call me.

"You don't need that stress," he told me. "But if it's necessary, we'll make it work," I said.

The Kincaids of Arlington, Virginia

In February, I started booking medical appointments starting the fourth week of April. That meant I would drive to Michigan to pick Mother and Dad up in a large, very comfortable rental car the week before. The key appointment, Doc Hall had said, should be with an oncology hematologist. I got recommendations. Yet, it wasn't really registering with me. Oncology.

My physicians were part of a health maintenance organization (HMO), with which I was completely unimpressed. So I wanted to stay far away from that organization. I called around and got recommendations from folks who were well versed in aging in Arlington County. One geriatrician was not taking new patients, so I decided to try more recent medical school graduates.

I decided on a woman physician for Mother and a man for Dad. Both were superb choices and restored my faith in the medical profession.

Then the move was scheduled. After medical week in Virginia, I was to return to Michigan to pack up household items and load the moving van.

The plan was coming together. The addition was on schedule for the April move-in date. Yet I knew my father's heart was breaking. He was upbeat when I talked with him because he knew Mother's health required the move, but he was much more anchored emotionally to the home he and Mother had built forty years earlier at the edge of St. Louis. Home was a place of significance to a man who was almost an orphan as a teenager. He still was connected to good friends and neighbors.

In one of my earlier visits, Dad suggested that I come back to Michigan to live. In the apartment attached to the house. Since I did so much work on my computer anyway, why wouldn't that work? It was unsaid; he didn't want to leave his home. I understood, but I couldn't run a business from 700 miles away. Later I heard him on the phone with a friend. "It didn't work," he reported. I pretended not to hear or understand. It just couldn't happen that way. Sadly.

As Mother's friends died, Alzheimer's tightened its vice on my mother's circle of support. A gregarious, chatty person, my mother had become more and more isolated by her disease, unable to reach out to make new friends.

The azaleas were in bloom in Virginia, I reported to my father just before I left. "Good, Mother will think they are for her," Dad said. Off I went on April 20, 2004.

As we packed up enough clothes to get my eighty-year old kids through two weeks and prepared for the drive to Virginia, the driveway filled with cars at 7 a.m. The Fab Four and Ann Hall came to sing Mother and Dad off for their new adventure. Ann had a camera and Mother and Dad listened as the pick-up quartet sang a couple of songs. It was a happy, thoughtful send-off, which would also serve to remind my dad how much he was leaving behind.

The wonderful photo of the Fab Four and Mother and Dad showed Mother without her glasses, and we ended up leaving her glasses behind.

As we left the house after the send-off, Mother was happy to be going on a car ride. Yet for Dad, the departure was filled with painful emotion. He sobbed the whole hour to Lansing. I understood his loss, or thought I did. Now, I wonder if I underestimated it.

I wrote later to family explaining the photo from that day. The guys in the pick-up quartet were the members of Team Kincaid, the Fab Four from Barbershoppers, who had become the lifeline—especially for my father over the last four years.

A bittersweet departure and a car filled with mixed emotion. Mother, happy to GO anywhere. Me, happy that the plan was coming together and optimistic that I could remove some of my father's caregiving burden. Dad, deeply mourning his loss of place and friends. Straight through to Arlington, our final destination. That was the plan and it worked.

*

Our Michigan neighbors, Deb and Dave Zimmerman, were buying

the house, and they were also doing the auction of its remaining contents. Dave said Dad helped him get a job early on that gave him a good start, though Dad didn't remember doing it.

Despite my efforts at strained cheerfulness, Dad's health was precarious. After Dad's second pneumonia bout in Arlington, there was a referral to a pulmonary group that was quite an experience.

There I was looking at the address, saying, "This can't be the place." But it was. So, I rolled the kids, age 88 and 87, out of the car. My dad was so frail he was in a portable wheelchair. We found our way to the reception room. Full of people. The reception desk staff could not be bothered to make eye contact. Now I was annoyed. "At least have the courtesy to have a conversation," I mumbled to myself. But it was not to happen.

No one in the reception room spoke. It was as though there was a cloud just before a storm over the energy level. Passive hostility was the message. We waited and waited. Finally, I had to leave my mother in the reception room and push my dad's wheelchair through what amounted to wheelchair barricades. Up and down. Sharp turn. Narrow doorway. Who in blazes designed this miserable space? Answer: no one. Dare I ask? Americans with Disabilities (ADA) compliance?

Not a chance. So, Dad and I arrived at the room with testing equipment. The hair on the back of my neck started to stand up. Better check on Mother. Back I went through the rabbit hutch to the reception room.

My mother was GONE. The Alzheimer's patient was missing.

To say I broke the silence of the reception desk was an understatement. Outside the office in the main lobby of this unsuitable medical facility, I found Mother. Rather quickly as a matter of fact. There she was sitting by the window looking at the trees. She didn't like the energy of the reception room and she was right. So very right. It was a miserable place so she up and left. Whew! I interjected a direct request to one of the queens on the front desk to ask if she could please keep an eye on my Alzheimer's patient. The crack staff. Now, at last, I seemed to have their attention.

*

On the health front, in addition to pneumonia, Dad had fluid on his lungs and four blood transfusions, and he learned to dislike overnights in Virginia Hospital Center. He enjoyed the outpatient transfusion center a lot, though. Our primary care doctors' offices and the hospital were only four minutes from the house. They knew us at valet parking.

Mother had done very well on Aricept, one of the older dementia/Alzheimer's medications; her new neurologist wanted to increase the dose, and in three months add Namenda, which was one of the medications now available for mid-to-severe dementia.

When the kids arrived in Arlington, I had in mind that we would have all of these fun-filled events. Didn't quite work out that way. Dad's health continued to decline. In addition to his weekly infusion at the hematologist, his blood counts were often so low that he had to be hospitalized.

We did mini-adventures: drove by the World War II memorial as it prepared for opening ceremonies; drove by my old house in Severna Park, Maryland; drove by an uncle and aunt's former house in Baltimore; and through Washington's many suburbs and surrounding areas.

One weekend party was particularly fun for all of us. My friend, Lynne, her daughter, Katie, Katie's husband Robert, and their four-year-old son Logan happened to be in the DC area in July. So I put together a brunch and invited my long-time friend, Tito, and his cousin who was in town from Italy.

My dad had grown very fond of Katie when she was a youngster. The Sells family and I both lived in the Annapolis area during the same period of time. Katie sometimes stayed with me when she needed a sitter. On this particular day, she was feeling poorly. She came to my house while my mother and father were helping me re-do the kitchen. My dad thought Katie was very mature and special. She had to be all of six at the time, quietly dropping her crab pot off the dock and watching it from her resting place near the living room window.

As a young mother, she was still special. At brunch Dad sat beside Katie. I have a photo of my dad from that brunch and he looked like a man who didn't have much time left. In fact, it turned out he died less than a month later.

Still, we had so much fun. Laughing and carrying on... Mother was terribly interested in Logan, the four-year-old. Good food. Great camaraderie.

After the brunch was over my dad said, "Now, that was a gathering of quality people." He was right, of course. There was nothing like long-time friends with shared personal histories. One rarely needed to explain anything.

My dad went into his room and I heard him talking on the phone. He had called Dave Zimmerman, who was handling the estate sale in Michigan. There was a toy truck that he wanted pulled from the sale so that he could give it to Logan.

Weeks later as my dad was dying in the hospital, the truck arrived. Still later at Christmas, I sent the truck to Katie for Logan. It was my dad's last present to anyone.

The months between April and August were more of a blur than I would like them to be. My father was dying. Some of the time I could feel that approaching reality. Other times I was fighting as hard as I could to keep him alive. Acknowledging what was likely ahead would have sapped my energy.

After one particularly miserable illness, my dear, dear father rested in bed and sobbed that he wanted to die. I felt as though I had been hit by a truck. He was the one who had taught me to push on, to fight for what I believed in. And now...

With some pride he would explain that when he was born he weighed two and a half pounds, was jaundiced, and not expected to live. The attending doctor was Dr. Hiram Winters. "If he lives," the doctor had said, "name him after me." So, my father used his middle name, Hiram, all of his life.

But now he was a man at the end of his life and not enjoying the misery of his health. His health made him feel useless. And, he was a man who needed to feel engagement and usefulness. I needed to listen CAREFULLY to his wishes. No assumptions. Hear his wishes. *Remember, you are HIS advance person!*

It was getting harder and harder to find foods he wanted to eat. Poached egg for breakfast was beginning to be our special time together. Fixing his egg, I would look at him and know that I wanted to remember the time together. I would touch his shoulder as I served him. No words were necessary. I was sure he understood. I don't remember where Mother was then. Not at the table, maybe still in bed, maybe looking out the front window.

Grant and Delores Colthorp from St. Louis came to visit. It was a farewell visit with my father, but I was pretending not to notice. As Grant stood to leave, my dad hugged him and told him he loved him. Later Grant would remember himself as the kid who arrived at the dry cleaners looking for a job. He got the job and a father figure for life. More than fifty years later, he would hear the words he had waited for all that time... my dad said, "I love you."

Those words didn't come easily. My dad had a wonderful bond with his two remaining siblings, Ron and Joan, who had been so very young when his mother died that both thought of themselves as orphans. Joan in her love of family had taught my dad to say, "I love you."

In those days, Mother was almost an afterthought. She was getting her meds regularly, but most of my energy was focused on the person who was more ill. Increasingly, Dad was not up to our driving adventures, but he encouraged me to take Mother. He would stay home and watch golf on television from his chair. I came to learn that "go" was a magical word for my Alzheimer's patient. Mother and I would launch one of our driving adventures out Route 66. Then we'd take the back roads and wander through the exquisite Virginia countryside to Middleburg. Stop for an ice cream and head back home. In the early and middle stages of Alzheimer's, car rides and ice cream were magical cures for agitation and repetitions, not to mention my anxiety.

In between patient care for both parents, I tried to work. Whenever I sat down at the computer, my mother would appear and start talking. I was frustrated and unpleasant. I even tried to figure out ways to lock her out of my space. Eventually, I just started working later at night after she had gone to bed. My dad was the one who wasn't sleeping; Mother was. They would sit and watch television together as they had for years. Old habits are often a good thing in Alzheimer's care. I found with Mother that the old habits of civility and courtesy helped to make life bearable in the early and middle stages.

Mother and Dad's sixty-fifth anniversary was Sunday, August 8. This day was August 2. Over the din of my television that night, I heard something. Sure enough, it was my father calling. He was in pain, terrible pain. This had started earlier in the day, but was clearly getting worse. Was it myelodysplastic syndrome turning to leukemia? All I had for pain was Tylenol. Celebrex had helped but the medication was now viewed as a danger. I was afraid to give him Celebrex. Did he want to go to the ER or wait until morning to call his doctor? Wait 'til morning, he decided. None of us slept, but we rested until morning.

Dad's doctor said he would meet us in the ER. We got Dad to the wheelchair and into the car and Mother and I took him there. The doctor was in, but things didn't seem to be moving quickly. At one point, I heard through the curtain my father asking the doctor to advise him on end-of-life care. I gulped in disbelief. Surely not this time... Surely this trip would not be that serious.

We waited for a room and waited some more. His color was better. He was clearly responding to the medications and transfusions. At one point, I took Mother home and fed her. I brought some homemade bean soup and cornbread back for Dad. A room had become available.

"Well, if it's going to be my last meal, that's what I want," my dad quipped as he saw the soup. Okay. Mother and I went home for the night at 10 p.m. At 11 p.m., the phone rang. My father had been taken to the ICU.

The voice on the phone said I was welcome to come to the ICU at any time, including now. What a dilemma. Should I be with him or should I stay with Mother? That question would occur over and over in the days ahead. There was no easy answer.

We waited until morning to go to the ICU. Subconsciously I was shifting my concern to my mother. Dad spoke quietly. He had started to choke on the cornbread and bean soup, he said. Was his ability to swallow going? He seemed to doze. Then suddenly his body seized. Shock, something... I wasn't sure. The staff came running, concerned looks on their faces. No words to Mother and me, but that was certainly all right.

I had had my last conversation with my father. The hematologist delivered the report. He would not survive this hospitalization. There was a massive infection and antibiotics would continue for a while. As I made arrangements for hospice, he was moved to a regular hospital room. Mother and I tried to keep a vigil. There was no extra bed or comfortable chair.

Every day Mother and I talked to him. I was sure he could hear even though he could no longer talk. Sunday, his 65th wedding anniversary, came. I told him the day. In my heart I believed he had resolved to stay alive for his 65th anniversary. I was sure.

Our vigil continued. I sensed that he and his body wanted to die, but that he also didn't want to leave us. Talk about dichotomy. Once I told him I was going to take Mother home. Then, I asked him to blink if he wanted me to stay. He blinked and I stayed another couple of hours. I decided to bring a boom box into the room. That way he could hear beautiful classical music even when we weren't there. Some comfort, I hoped. As I left each night to take Mother home, I obsessed that the people who cared for him would know who he was. He wasn't just some old man left there to die. People loved him. So, I put a copy of his life story on the window ledge for anyone who was curious.

In what felt very much like another moment of grace, the night nurse came on. Her compassion was clear. She saw his story, read it, and promised—volunteered actually—to keep the music playing overnight. I knew the end was near, but I really believed he would live through the night. He did.

The next morning around 11 o'clock, I noticed something different and walked to his side. "Daddy, Mother and I are here. We love you."

Then he took his final breath. Handel's "Hallelujah Chorus" played.

GRIEF: LOSING AND SORROW

The downside of loving has always been losing. I had been here before. My younger self used to try to hide from losing, recognizing early on the suffering and pain associated with loss. I still remember looking into that casket at the funeral home and seeing my dad's brother there. I was ten. And, I saw my father cry. I felt the same agony when I saw my father dead. He was the one person in my family who remembered my birthday. He was the one person who cared whether I got home from a trip safely. He was my partner in caring for my mother.

As a kid, the flowers, the traditional statement of comfort, gave me a headache. Only when I got the same headache when President Kennedy died years later did I realize that it was grief that made me physically ill, not the flowers.

Every now and then I try to think of all of the words that describe grief. Usually, I give up around the Ds: despair, distress. Even as a little kid I was preoccupied with sadness and sorrow. Of course, I didn't talk out loud about it. My fear was abandonment, becoming an orphan, being left alone. People in my dad's family were dying young from a hereditary disease. If I talked about it, I would make people, especially Mother and Dad, uncomfortable. "Good people" didn't make others uncomfortable. It wasn't nice, and people wouldn't like you if you weren't nice. Besides, they were exhausted from their work, and sharing my angst with them would only make them more tired. I held those views until I was fifty at least. *Hmm, maybe thirty.*

There was a lot to grieve for as a caregiver. The personal life I gave up for ten years, dinners and evenings with friends. Movies, theater, and concerts. A significant other. The professional life I gave up. Oddly, I never felt specific grief for any of those. Some people feel that a lot. I didn't. I think I compartmentalized it. Did I suppress it? Not quite, I think. *Later*, I thought. *I'll get back to it again. Not now.* Yet, I knew there was an underlying grief in my being. Sadness and sorrow could come very quickly. Only occasionally was it severe. When I was ill, I was most aware. There I was, back to that childhood fear. Who would take care of me if I couldn't?

It's so hard to find the right words. Grief was kind of dormant, lying inside like the chicken pox virus, ready to pop out unexpectedly as an altered disease. Yet, more like a composite of all the losses than a singular virus like shingles.

Stages of grief are an inadequate explanation when you're inside them. Suggestions that "he/she's in a better place," never cut it with me. The Warrior Princess wanted to scream, "And how do you know?" The deceased didn't check in after death. Seriously, there is no evidence. Yes, I'd like to believe it, but just don't say that to me and expect me to be immediately comforted. It doesn't work for me. Maybe that's what started me writing. Looking for the right words to explain the upheaval, disorientation, and sense of lost control. Not to mention lost hope.

Practice makes reading, writing, riding a bicycle—most things— easier. Not my experience with grief. Oh, there's a muscle memory factor. In my experience, it seems to compound the process, making it more difficult. The weight and burden of previous sorrows are remembered as fresh and new. All of them over again. Not the recovery or the healing that eventually softens the blows. The nonstop dreams of loss. The sense of no control. The feelings of failure. That's my immediate muscle memory. Eventually, the degree of discomfort softens, but the memories remain and the dreams are exhausting.

When it softens, it isn't the first thing you think of when you wake up. Maybe it's the third or fourth. Eventually, you don't think about it until noon. And, so on. But, loss is there. As it softens, I may be more able to put one foot in front of the other. I may be less dysfunctional, but I still remember the loss and feel a sense of melancholy.

We are so weird about grief and death.

Afterlife is another contradictory subject for me. Part of me likes the idea of being able to flit around as a spirit after I die. I want to hang out with people I like. Another part of me rejects meeting family and friends in some, vague cosmic afterlife. How is it organized? Do you take a number when you arrive? How do you find your family members in the midst of all of the other people? Zip codes? Cell phones? Do you sit or lie down? Lying down would be my preference. I wouldn't mind sleeping a lot. The organizational aspect of an afterlife is something I just can't get a handle on and organization is a big deal for me. I'm a Virgo.

*

Intellectually, I think I will be accepting of my own death. I say that, but I recognize that I'm not ready yet. Also, I will be furious about the disease that gets me. It's hard to imagine that I will go quietly. Accepting, but furious. Another contradiction? Well, yes. Isn't everything?

MOTHER AND ME—2004

Kincaid Cousin Bob Arnott flew in from Denver to drive Mother and me to West Virginia for Dad's funeral. I was pretty much a blithering idiot. Grant Colthorp, Dad's longtime friend and also a pastor in Michigan, came to do the service.

Mother and I went home alone. It was eerie. I, who had often been the one who didn't cry much, could barely see through the tears to get out of town. Too much emotion in my being and my eyes. But, I cried secretly; I didn't want my mother to know. My mother, dry-eyed, quietly enjoyed the landscape of her homeland. As we drove by the cemetery, I worried whether my father was cold on this steaming hot August day. Four months earlier, I was so happy when we arrived in Virginia. I could help my father and he would live longer. Already, I had failed. He did not live longer. He was gone in what seemed like no time.

I needed a new plan. We were two now. I absolutely had to increase my focus on work even though my father—my sitter and best helper with Mother's care—was gone.

About a week after we returned from West Virginia, Mother said, "I miss Hiram."

I had been wondering how much she remembered. We were sitting in my bedroom. There was sadness about us, even though I pushed to stay busy with errands that had been delayed.

Then we talked for a while about how much we missed him. I cried. She didn't. Before Alzheimer's, she always cried.

"I feel so lonely," she said. "I want to stay close. I want *US* to stay close."

"We will," I reassured her.

"I didn't want him to stay like that," she said, referring to his last days in the hospital, unable to swallow or talk. I was reminded of her comment in the hospital room. Before the morgue came for the body, I asked her if she wanted to go. "No," she said. "He's mine and I'm staying."

Sometimes, she hardly knew she was married to him. But other times she knew absolutely. That she loved him and that he took care of her. Sometimes she thought he was her brother or her father. But this day, she was crystal clear about her loss and who he was. Those were the moments that made family caregiving for me. If we could have afforded assisted living and she would have lived there, I might have missed these small, occasional moments of lucidity. So meaningful.

Her sense of my father was similar to her sense of who I was. Sometimes, she thought I was one of her sisters, Lucille or Lenore. She might call me Barbara, but she talked to me about Barbara as though she was unable to connect the idea that I was Barbara, her daughter.

For me the sadness of my lost father was ever present and my mourning delayed. At night, the same dream kept coming over and over. I would just get to sleep. The phone would ring. It was the ICU telling me my father was there and I could come to visit anytime. But, of course, my mother was sleeping in the next room. I couldn't leave her. Over and over, the grinding guilt of not being there.

*

Earlier, Mother and I had gone for an intake interview at an adult day care center in Fairfax County. Dad was still alive. I was finding my way as a family caregiver. The center was a well-regarded service provider that was fee-for-service. At the time I was thinking about sending Mother a couple of days a week, which would have cost about $70 a day. My father, the thrifty Scotsman, rejected the center based on cost.

I had to admit that he was right, given our financial picture. Our interview wasn't exactly a winner, either. The nurse got up close and personal with Mother. In her face and a little too *loud*. Some providers believe with older folks you just talk louder and more slowly. Miss Dixie was not hard of hearing. Once the staffer turned her back, Miss Dixie turned to me and mumbled, "That didn't do a thing for me." I chuckled and agreed.

Later, I learned about a county-run adult day care program in

Arlington. Although it was not explicitly a program for Alzheimer's patients, Mother would be eligible for it in the early to mid-stages of her disease. But, the real beauty was that fees were sliding scale based on income, and my mother's income was low. My mother's daily rate was a little under $16. I was elated.

On the way to the intake interview with my mother, I told her about the activities. Art, music, games, and small group discussions. Field trips to see the leaves in the fall or flowers in the spring. Celebrations for Mardi Gras, St. Patrick's Day, Halloween, and all the major holidays. Breakfast, lunch, and snacks. And, maybe friends. "Like school," she interrupted at one point. "Yes, like school," I responded. I knew it would work when she said school. She would like it!

Much earlier when I had tried to get her interested in an Alma program, she was adamant that she was not going. No way! What changed? I don't know completely. But, she was deeper into her disease so her previous objections were forgotten. And clearly I was learning how to frame ideas for her, too. The truth of the matter was that there was not going to be a choice of her going or not going now. I needed to work, but there was no point in presenting it to her that way. Alas, I was beginning to learn that Alzheimer's patients, like the rest of us, don't like to be bossed around either.

*

Our intake interview at the Madison Center, a former Arlington elementary school, was with the social worker. The interview went well, and that's where Mother became Miss Dixie. It was really who she was as an Alzheimer's patient—an odd combination of propriety with an edge. (The edge came when she kicked and hit, as her disease advanced.) Miss Dixie started adult day care with three days. We went quickly to four and five. Transportation was available, but I chose to drive her.

Caregivers like me first came to day care for respite care, but the word "respite" was a misnomer. Yes, I was looking for an opportunity to earn a living, to go to the dentist, and other necessary healthcare appointments. As I came to learn, there were more important reasons for Miss Dixie and others who spent time playing bingo, bowling, and golf. These activities could engage and reward. They provided a sense of belonging and socialization that was otherwise missing for the Alzheimer's patient. I had actually tried to organize some excursions to the Botanic Garden, art galleries, and art classes at home for the weeks before our intake interview. All were things she loved at one time, but not now. It was a bust, perhaps because it was just the two of us. It lacked the sense of community that she came to enjoy in her own little world at day care.

A lovely white-haired woman named Margaret seemed to become Mother's friend at day care. Margaret was in a wheelchair and did not have dementia. She was a sunny, happy woman.

Miss Dixie was chatty and social before Alzheimer's. Even though several friends were younger than Mother, I remembered a poignant conversation from before Alzheimer's set in, when her last friend died. With a very matter-of-fact tone, my mother said, "My last friend is gone." It's hard enough to find true friends without the confusion and memory loss of Alzheimer's. Pretty much impossible with Alzheimer's. Besides, her husband of sixty-five years was gone now, too.

In a holiday fundraising letter in 2005, I asked other family caregivers to join me with a charitable gift to Madison Center with the following:

"Like you, I suspect, I worry about money all of the time. It is terrifying to contemplate a worst-case scenario. But one of the lessons I am trying to learn from my mother is that life is a lot easier if you focus on today. *Today, I am enormously grateful to the staff and volunteers of the Madison Center.* I am also grateful to the wonderful people who have become my mother's friends at Madison Center... possibly your mother or father. So, my gift is really a small token of appreciation to everyone who makes up the community of Madison Center.

"Thank you for your kindness and caring. Thank you for making my mother smile..."

The new opportunities for socialization were the first bonus I noticed. A chat with Margaret quickly became part of our daily afternoon pick-up scenario. I looked forward to seeing Margaret, and she would fill me in on their activities. Then, Margaret wasn't there. Probably the flu, I thought. I asked about her after a week or so. The answer I received?

She died. In the world of caring for seniors, sudden loss was part of my own learning curve.

I enjoyed others at day care. One man who was clearly interested in

Mother came up to me as I was picking her up. "Bet she was a looker in her day," he said and sort of asked at the same time.

"Yes," I said. "Yes, she was." Weeks later I saw him at a skilled nursing facility with his wife. *I'm sure he just forgot he had a wife. Happens with dementia.*

Another exchange with a very sweet woman happened after Mother had been away for a few days.

"Dixie talked today," the woman said. I guess she hadn't been talking much at day care. "She told me she liked my shoes." I could pick up all kinds of information with my daily trips to and from day care.

On the way to day care one morning, Mother told me that it made her so happy to see my father's smile first thing in the morning and the last thing at night. I positioned, quite by accident, a favorite photo of the two of them in his sitting room just off their bedroom. The picture was taken on their sixty-fourth wedding anniversary. Before Alzheimer's my mother would have been crippled with grief by his death and would not have been able to feel anything but disabling sorrow. When her sister, Lucille, died Mother stopped painting for two years. So, in this peculiar way, I was enormously grateful for her disease. She knew Dad was gone, but her customary sorrow had been dulled by her disease.

The Healing Power of Being Heard

Not long ago, I looked up the word "support" in an Internet dictionary and one of the definitions seemed on target for Alzheimer's family caregiver support groups.

"To keep from weakening or failing; strengthen..." In other words, to help a caregiver endure the long and arduous crossing that was Alzheimer's.

After Dad's death, and once I got Miss Dixie settled into day care, I looked for a new caregiving support group. Groups run by volunteers were sponsored by the Alzheimer's Association and listed on the local chapters' website. The evening groups I used to attend no longer worked now that I was a sole caregiver, 24/7.

Twice a month a group met in Arlington during the day while Miss Dixie was in day care. This time would work. Would I feel an affinity to the group? What I did feel was a certain amount of anxiety as I wandered into to the community room as the new person. Two large tables were set up in a corner of the room. The gathering was dwarfed, almost minimized by the size of the room. People had pieces of paper folded like tents as identifiers. First names were scrawled in black marker ink. I made my tent and wrote my name. Other groups that I attended had been in small conference rooms of long-term care facilities. Those were more intimate, but I was open to seeing how this one worked.

The facilitator, a former caregiving husband whose wife had died a couple of years earlier, was likeable and charming. He had a Southern accent and a good sense of humor.

Five or six people spoke about what was going on with their Alzheimer's person: wife, husband, parent, boyfriend, sister. Each story was different, painful in its distinctive way. It sounded as though they had all been caregiving a long time.

Then, it was my turn. I said my name and started to cry. I couldn't stop. I told my story in tears and between sobs. I was surprised, but oddly I wasn't embarrassed. Later I learned that people have often cried on that first visit. The thing that surprised me most was that it was NOT my first visit to a support group. It was my first time with THIS group, yes, but for four years I had attended other groups. Now, however, I was a sole family caregiver. I had never cried before.

Why did I cry—sob, really—on this first visit? I'm not sure I'll ever know. Relief? Release? Probably. As good an explanation as any, I guess.

As I returned to the group, I began to learn more. One mantra was: *If you've seen one case of Alzheimer's, you've seen ONE case.* And a second: *The caregiver's health and wellbeing was as important as the patient's.* Then, I started learning from individual stories. Lucinda, white-haired, petite, and young-looking, was caring for her boyfriend and life partner. Her father also had dementia, probable Alzheimer's, and was further along. He was beginning to be violent. Lucinda was concerned about her mother as his primary caregiver.

Alfred's wife, Patricia, had early onset Alzheimer's. Her symptoms became noticeable in her early sixties. Both were world travelers and singers. Alfred, a law school professor, noticed her symptoms as Patricia's trip preparation skills went downhill. Her disease progressed rapidly and she was in a small assisted living home now. At one point she had been admitted to hospice care, but then she improved and the unit released her. Still, her condition was worsening. Weekend drives and singing together were no longer possible. She was bedridden, and the determined and kind nursing aide kept her alive by feeding her one tiny sip at a time.

Marta was looking after her sister, who lacked other immediate family. In a nursing home, her sister's anger made Marta's visits several times a week sad. Her Alzheimer's was advanced and she was often agitated, angry, and violent. The nursing home used Seroquel, one of the antipsychotic medications, to sedate her, but finding the right dosage was a circus of frustration for Marta. In a cruel stroke of irony, Marta's husband started displaying memory problems after her sister's death. But even more cruel was that Marta herself seemed headed down that path, after anesthesia for a major surgery started affecting her.

All were new friends by virtue of the journey we were on. There was something special and almost magical about this particular group. I have often made modest reference to these people as the "world's greatest support group." The folks who attend come and go, but the spirit of the mutual respect has stayed. Smart, articulate people talked honestly and openly about what was going on in their respective lives and how they felt about it. Pretenders and drama queens and kings generally didn't stay long. Authenticity was part of the glue that connected us.

However, it was difficult to articulate the bond. Once we had a newcomer who said, "You people all sound like you know each other." We did know each other, but only from sharing our Alzheimer's experience for an hour and a half, twice a month.

Confidentially was an underlying principal, but it was measured against the importance of telling the story of Alzheimer's. Pain, sorrow masked as anger, frustration with the patient, with doctors, with aides and care managers who made promises they didn't deliver, sorrow, guilt, sorrow. Who was really good! Who was so-so! Who to call if you were absolutely at the end of your rope. We understood to the extent that anyone could understand another's experience. Respect and the belief that each person's journey was distinct and different were part of the unspoken code. If we had experienced something similar we shared it, but we always tried to honor the differences of each experience. A humorous story was saved for group, for these special people who would get it quickly and laugh boldly, as though it was therapy—because it was. Just as people said cruel and unthinking things to the bereaved, they also said ridiculous things to caregivers. It was hard not to scream. Not to respond as rudely and invasively as his or her words.

The collective knowledge of the group was useful. Who were the quality psychiatrists for geriatric patients; the internists who could relate to dementia patients? What medications could a caregiver request for psychotic episodes? Who were the geriatric care managers who, for a consulting fee, could help plot a care plan with the appropriate services, based on individual resources, etc.? What facilities would take Medicaid if one was close to needing that? On and on.

Perhaps most importantly, each looked at the other and said with kindness and credibility, "You are important, too. You have to take care of yourself or you will be doing no good for anyone."

Why do support groups work? So often we heard someone say,

"Well, at least I don't have THAT to deal with..." How could you not feel a little better about your own situation! The group helped caregivers tap into creative solutions. It also helped set parameters for trial and error tactics. The only given in Alzheimer's care was the need for constant readjustment. Every day was a craps shoot. Sometimes all that was needed was to be HEARD when other professionals, who should have been listening, didn't seem to be.

Not every group works, but finding a good group is like striking gold. Value beyond description.

STORIES FROM THE GROUP

Each Alzheimer's story is and was different. Stories from the Arlington caregiving support group illustrate the differences. Names have been changed and permission to tell each story has been granted.

One wonderful spouse slept at the top of the stairs to be certain that her clever, crafty husband didn't escape into the dark of night. She found gifts in the form of fecal matter under the furniture in the living room, and there was often a trail of incontinence as they left a store. And yes, she knew the benefit of regularly scheduled bathroom visits. Sometimes tactics worked and sometimes they didn't.

Another person went missing for two days. One of the issues that I struggled with and that my friend, Lucinda, struggled with was allowing the patient as much independence and freedom as the patient's condition would allow. Finding the balance with Alzheimer's could be difficult; what the patient could do safely one day, the next day he or she could not. It happened without warning. Lucinda's Jerry was living alone, caring for himself and his pets, and walking daily. Living safely. Then, he wasn't.

One Saturday, Jerry disappeared on his walk. GONE. The police were notified. The search included friends, flyers, newspaper articles, a helicopter, and a bloodhound. Quite by accident, Jerry was found asleep on the street, thirteen miles from his home. What happened and how he got there was never known, of course. Lucinda's next move was to interview and select a live-in, twenty-four hour caregiver, since she had decided that Jerry had the resources to stay in his own home as long as possible.

One of the things Lucinda suffered was guilt. From time to time we all felt guilt. Guilt that you didn't see "it" coming, whatever "it" was. Freedom was one of the great losses that dementia patients sustained.

The freedom to be, to come and go as one pleased, to eat what and when one wanted. Those things all disappeared with dementia, and humane caregiving put us right at the brink of making those choices for the patient. Anyone who allowed as much freedom as could be had without danger to the patient always ran a risk. I believed the risk was worth taking, but I knew it was a difficult choice.

One of the men who cared for his wife moved into the Alzheimer's unit of an assisted living facility to provide comfort and companionship, as he had done throughout their decades of marriage. His love and concern and cheerfulness was a wonderful example for all. Not long after her death, he moved back to an independent living apartment, and recently he found a new companion/partner.

Another man developed a creative solution to his wife's repetitive demands that he take her home. She was already home, of course, but he helped her put her coat on, turned out the lights, and drove around the block so that she could happily return to where she lived. *Hey, it worked.* Sadly, he died during a brief hospitalization before his wife, who was then in a nursing home.

Unable to handle the outbursts in home care, especially directed at her in-home caregivers, another man reluctantly moved his wife to a specialized care facility, which he visited several times a day. The new environment worked much better for some reason. Though the common perception was that staying home was desirable, it did not work well in this case. Who knew why home care didn't work? It just didn't.

Jocelyn's husband was diagnosed with early onset Alzheimer's that took hold of their lives while both were in their fifties. A government lawyer, he began having trouble at work. His disease progressed rapidly and Jocelyn had a home health aide come in several days a week. Hallucinations and violent protective actions became part of his pattern. Jocelyn hid the kitchen knives, but he threatened the health aide with a frying pan and ripped the shower curtain down trying to protect himself from a helper in the shower. After a fall, he was hospitalized briefly, and that was the point at which Jocelyn moved him to a small assisted living home. He settled in quickly without additional "calming" medication. Jocelyn believed his adjustment to his new surroundings was helped by behaving as a guest would. The power of guest behavior! Who knew!

Harriett, an elder-care lawyer, found that she had to divorce her second husband, the Alzheimer's patient, in order to restore a veteran's benefit. Part of the issue was protecting assets for three special needs children from her first marriage. Still, she had her ex-husband's medical power of attorney, went to court after the divorce to be made his guardian, and remained committed to his care and end-of-life decisions. She was with him when he died. His children were grateful for her presence and care.

Margaret was in her second decade as a long-distance caregiver for two parents who were separated. Her father was dead now, but she had managed her parents' care using different yet creative approaches for each parent. While her father had been cared for in a nursing home, a care manager and team of six part-time assistants helped Margaret's mother in northwestern Pennsylvania. Each assistant had different activity assignments. One assistant who liked to sing took her mother to choir practice; another took her to bingo. A third walked with her several times a week. The anxiety of not being on-site as illnesses arose was highly stressful, but Margaret's mother seemed to do very well in her own house with lots of supporting services.

Group member Sybil offered an explanation of the changes a spouse felt as Alzheimer's entered her relationship with her wonderful husband Bob, a highly decorated Navy pilot who looked like he'd come straight from central casting.

"I think of him as my third husband," she explained. "He's not the person I fell in love with as my second husband. There are some similarities, but he's different. So, he's my third."

*

One of my favorites was a man several called Eisenhower. No, not "Ike." That was too informal. He had an Army general's bearing because he was one: a retired two-star major general. I discovered that only when I googled him. He had a quiet presence, and I was curious. As we learned years later, he was also an extraordinary hero from World War II. But, we met him in his nineties as a caregiver for his wife Ann. Like everyone else in the group, we called him by his first name.

Eisenhower came to group in a sports jacket and tie, along with his son, who had slipped away from a busy office to support his father in his caregiving. (Most of us wore retirement casual.) Eisenhower's wife was a mid-to-late stage Alzheimer's patient. At one point, Ann had opened the passenger door of the car. The car was moving. Now, he was caring for her in various assisted living facilities. Though the facilities had good reputations, there was something seriously unsatisfactory about each.

Here was a man in his nineties who had more mental and physical capacity than most forty-year-old law partners. He was awakened in the middle of the night by a nursing aide, checking to see if his pants were dry. Groans erupted from the group when we heard this report. Was this intrusion really necessary? Over the period of time that we knew Eisenhower, there were typical ups and downs with Alzheimer's care.

One of the many memorable traits Eisenhower displayed was his continued respect for Ann, who was also a retired Army major. During one difficult period, he told us he was waiting and hoping that his wife would have a good day so he could discuss a new care option with her. He was reluctant to make a decision that involved her unilaterally.

Like others in the group, Eisenhower found institutional policies frequently ran counter to what he considered in the best interest of his wife's care. At one point, he was certain she needed to be moved from a nursing home bed to the hospital, and he had reached his limit of patience.

He spoke quietly but firmly as he put it this way: "You have three minutes before I call 911. The time starts now," he said, as he looked at his watch.

She went to the hospital. He was still a man of decisive presence.

After Ann died, he called to say he was sorry to miss one of our Christmas parties and to tell us a little about what he had been doing. In his nineties, he was still looking to improve his swimming stroke. He had found a coach, he reported. Already he was an extraordinary swimmer setting national and international records in his age group.

Indeed, swimming and heroism had earned him the Distinguished Service Cross in World War II. He was leading a battalion south of Paris on the Seine River, and across the river the Germans were in a heavily fortified position. The bridges were impassable and US Army assault boats were delayed behind Allied lines. There was no support to count on. Despite the circumstances, the US objective was to build a pontoon bridge. Eisenhower noticed a line of five rowboats on the other side of the river. He took off his uniform and boots and swam the river. Then he released the lead boat that was tied to a stake. All five boats were connected and he pulled them across the river. Somehow, the Germans missed this maneuver, perhaps believing that no one would dare such a move. After American troops and guns secured the bank, the borrowed boats were used to prepare the pontoon bridge.

Later, at the Village of Dornot on the Moselle River, Eisenhower's battalion sustained heavy losses but heroically battled the Germans so that another pontoon bridge could be successfully built. In conversations about this time, the general remembered it as the most difficult communication he ever made to his troops. It was clear that without additional support, heavy casualties would be the outcome.[13] Yet, the battle was to continue as a distraction for another Allied crossing south at Arnaville, which was viewed by command as strategically more important. The village square in Dornot was named for our friend in 2009, a year after Ann died. All four of his children and their families attended the dedication. Our distinguished friend died in his hundredth year, a few months short of his birthday. An extraordinary human being and example for all of us in so many ways.

Each group meeting had new stories and new twists to caregiving. At some point almost all caregivers, including me, verbalized sorrow, resentment, worry, fear, anger, isolation, and guilt. But the saving grace was there, too. "At least I don't have THAT to deal with," was always close to the surface as one listened to others.

---

13. "French Villages Hail a Liberator," *Village Voice* (Asbury), November/December, 2009.

SWEETNESS AND CHARM

Looking back, the middle stage of Alzheimer's was not terribly complicated for Miss Dixie and me. It did not seem to be the case at the time, of course. But there was a daily pattern and schedule emerging. There were car rides. We could go to restaurants and on shopping errands together. She could get in and out of the car by herself, in and out of bed, and explore the house on her own. I once heard her talking to someone at the front of the house. When I went to see what was happening, she was having an animated conversation in the mirror with herself. Judging from her facial expression, it was a good talk.

Another time, she rolled out of bed with her shoes on. "Why?" I asked. "Well, I don't want to lose them." Losing her shoes had certainly become an issue. She would get out of bed independently and hide her shoes, forgetting afterward that she had done anything. They might be stuffed between the mattress and the springs on her bed, or in the closet, or in another room.

And *my* shoes. If I made the mistake of leaving them outside the door of my small bathroom, my shoes would disappear while I took a shower.

Once, as we walked through a department store, she stopped dead in her tracks. A baby in a stroller had her full attention. "Well, aren't you precious!" she told the baby with a big smile on her face. The child's mother beamed, even though she didn't speak English.

The waiter at the local diner recognized us and called me by name when we made our monthly visit, while the cleaning person was finishing up at home.

Mother was pleasant to be around, and friends were kind to invite both of us to holiday parties. "Who is she?" a friend asked, pointing to me.

"My mother," Miss Dixie replied. *Okay, I didn't say it was perfect.* She also knew she was supposed to say something when we left a beautiful house after a fabulous dinner. Her version of appreciation was, "We'll be back!"

We even went to a large summer lawn party near Charles Town, West Virginia. Great food, fiddle music, and dancing. This particular day was chilly so Miss Dixie borrowed a jacket. And, she had her straw hat on. I could swear I never left her side. As we were leaving, somehow, somehow, every pocket of that jacket got stuffed with cookies. Hands so quick...

At home as I took her hat off, a cloth napkin floated to the ground.

Silly me, I asked, "Where'd that come from?" Miss Dixie shrugged in her bewilderment. "Fell from the sky..."

Miss Dixie also developed her own games. I would help her into her side of the car. I hitched up her seat belt and moved the door so she could reach it enough to close it. I would get in the driver's side and see her shoulders hunch over with a little movement at the corner of her eye. Then, *bam.* Her game was to close her door at the same time I closed mine. She would turn and smile. Success was so sweet.

In the drive through at Wendy's, she quietly read the sign out loud. "Pick up WINDOW. I don't want a WINDOW."

"Okay," I said, smiling as I turned my head.

Even though Miss Dixie wore the Safe Return bracelets of the Alzheimer's Association, there was still the frightening possibility she could wander off. It was amazing how quickly she could disappear. Once I noticed that the house seemed really quiet. Did I lock the door? (All the locks had to be changed to keyed deadbolts, by the way.) No, I didn't, and she was gone. I jumped in the car and a block and a half away I found her huffing and puffing up a hill. Because she was tired, Miss Dixie was really happy to see me; forgetting, I presume, her reason for her adventure. She had put her hat on, of course. A necessity even when you were running away from home.

At this stage of Alzheimer's, her mobility was not impaired. As it got lighter in the summer months, I would occasionally find her sitting in her nightgown with her wet diaper on my good upholstered chairs in the living room, looking out the window. Other times I would find her diapers hidden in drawers, or with my architects' drawings wrapped around them. She had both independence and mobility, and no sense of appropriateness.

I found that I needed sitters, really companions at this stage, who could stay with her, talk to her, and keep her safe during an afternoon on the weekend or an evening. I sent an email to a local seminary for candidates from the student body. That worked well until the students got very busy. Then, I tried Craigslist online. It turned out to be a great source of sitter companions.

On the downside, though, every now and then I was met at day care with a report of kicking or hitting. I was never clear on the purpose of the report. I really couldn't talk to her about changing her behavior. That was part of the disease. *And the purpose of telling me was... ?*

At this point, there were minor changes in Miss Dixie's ability to function on her own, but that would begin to change.

THE COLLATERAL STUFF—2005

There we were, pretty much minding our own business when urinary tract infections (UTI) reared their heads. I was really dumb about the first one, and Miss Dixie couldn't tell me if she felt different. I had never had a UTI. Thank heavens for day care. The folks at Madison noticed that Miss Dixie was not her usual self. I had actually noticed that also, but I wasn't sure what the cause might be. The program director clued me in that I needed to have Mother checked for a urinary infection. It was the end of the week and I decided to do it first thing the next week.

Over the weekend, Miss Dixie got really sick. Waiting until Monday was no longer an option. I couldn't get her out of bed. I couldn't move her. So, I called an emergency medical service (EMS) to transport her. This was our first trip to the emergency room (ER) with Mother. We had visited several times with Dad, but I always took him by car with a borrowed portable wheelchair.

At the hospital, I arrived a few minutes after the ambulance and found her dozing but propped up in bed. I told the nurses and doctor that I was sure she had a urinary infection. So, they prepared for a test. Since she was unable to pee in a jar at that point, the nurse was to insert a catheter. I was surprised when the nurse asked me to leave. But, no problem. I left.

When I came back into the room, Miss Dixie was giving me the high sign. Her right eyebrow shot up in a scrunch. There was a look that I had seen many times over the years. A nod of her head also told me she wanted me to come closer to her bed. I was being summoned immediately. The look said, "Have I got something to tell you!"

In the meantime, the nurse was very pleasantly telling us how to get in touch with her if we needed her. I could see the look on Mother's face getting stormier and more urgent. Finally, the nurse left. I leaned my head in so mother could whisper her secret. *Okay, let's hear it, Miss Dixie.*

"She's a shit-ass," announced my mother.

I dropped my face into my hands so she wouldn't see me laugh. Her outrage was simple and direct. Her choice of words was atypical. She was really angry. *I guess the catheter procedure didn't go so well.* I rolled my eyes, took a deep breath, and faced her, changing the subject.

In the mid-stages of Alzheimer's, we were looking at lots of urinary infections on a yearly basis. At least six a year. At one point, I created our own three-step response to the issue. First, I traded her morning and evening juice from orange to "cranberry light." After one hospitalization, I happened onto very large diapers for nighttime. My theory was that the moisture would be further away from the tract and her skin. Then I started giving her a morning shower daily so that she could be washed thoroughly with running water every morning. Medical people recommended bathing a couple of times a week, but I felt our situation warranted more attention. We went a long time without an infection, but as her disease progressed we were dealing with about three a year. So my technique cut the incidence in half roughly. *Not bad for an amateur.*

*

I had decided that I needed to visit the cemetery in West Virginia where my father was buried. It was really important to me, and it had been almost a year since his death. I knew part of my emotional need resulted from a failure to grieve. Sure, I had cried, but I really hadn't worked through the pain. I had bottled it up. Too much to do. I decided that May 3—his birthday—would be the perfect time. There was a cheap flight from Dulles Airport to Charleston, so I thought about flying. I made plans, including getting a photo identification card for Mother. We sat at the Virginia Department of Motor Vehicles for a while, not too long really, and got her ID. Then, I decided to drive.

As the date approached, Mother picked up a terrible cold at day care and my plans fell apart. I was devastated at first. But the more I thought about it, I realized that Miss Dixie's cold saved us from my really crazy idea. Thinking that I could drive us to West Virginia was insane. I had lost my mind—temporarily, I hoped. I had wanted so much to visit the cemetery, but it was not to be.

After I adjusted to my disappointment at missing the West Virginia trip, I recognized that Mother's Alzheimer's had progressed significantly in the months since Dad's death. Too much to handle a seven-hour driving trip with uncertain rest stops. She was fine operating in our daily routine most of the time, but trying to take on a major adventure by myself made no sense at all. So, Miss Dixie's illness saved me from myself. That, or a helpful hand from Providence.

Later in the month, we received a call that her brother in Texas, Richard, had died. We had not known he was ill. A World War II pilot, he was next in birth order to Mother. One of the few photos of my mother's childhood was with Richard. In addition, he and my dad had been close friends in high school. Both played football and both ran for senior class president. My dad won. I felt a tremendous sense of loss that I was unable to share with Miss Dixie. I didn't tell her; she would not have understood. So much of family connections was based on shared memory. When they were gone, another loss of significant proportions.

*

Ups and downs in her care started to increase. The sniff-and-whiff test had become part of my bag tricks also. First, it was urine. Now it was fecal matter. *Nothing like a good strong whiff of incontinence to get your morning rolling. Ah, the distinct aroma...*

I tried not to jump to conclusions. I would ask myself, "Is it?" *Yes, I think it is.* Time to start the laundry machine and get the rubber gloves. Even a year into the hands-on care timeframe, I was trying to make do with my small washing machine that was efficient for a single person household, but inefficient for my current circumstances. A major incontinence bout meant five or six loads of laundry. Since I had a washing machine, I had not questioned its size. Once I was into caregiving, it became clear that a larger size would simplify my workload. *Another overlooked issue on my part.*

As usual, the thrift gene had reared its ugly head. I didn't have the space for a separate washer and dryer, so the price of a large combination machine would put me into a perpetual state of hyperventilation. After about six months of laundry hell, I broke down and bought a big honking machine. As I arrived at the decision, I managed to beat myself up. "How did Lucille do laundry for Grandmother?" I asked myself. *She drove miles to the laundromat, wimp.*

When I started using that big machine, I thought I had won the lottery, and I didn't care how much it cost. Funny how your perspective changes. I loved that big, ugly thing.

Betrayal, Exhaustion, and Respite Care

With encouragement from my support group, I began to think about respite care for two weeks at an assisted living facility. I had a new contract through my consulting business that theoretically might require travel, so I believed I needed to do a trial run in case the issue came up. A member of the support group was also on staff at an assisted living home. It had an appeal, since it looked like a large pleasant home inside and out. I was more comfortable with the idea of turning Miss Dixie's care over to someone else, since I knew a staff member and knew she had parents in New Jersey who were facing similar issues.

There were quite a few hoops to jump through to prepare for the respite. Another physical examination and tuberculosis inoculation needed to happen, despite the fact that Mother had had all of this less than a year ago in preparation for day care. I wasn't smart enough to challenge the inoculation necessity and I should have. She needed iron-on tags for her clothes, like a kid going to summer camp. I fretted about how she might sleep comfortably, since she was used to a bed that raised her back and feet to perfectly comfortable positions automatically. Now, for two weeks she would need to depend on pillows and someone remembering to adjust them. Was I throwing her into a risky situation without intending to? I really needed to explore this care option in case I needed to use it. So, this was a test run.

As I took Mother to assisted living for the two weeks, I thought I was having a nervous breakdown. For two weeks I had been a basket case, crying at the drop of a hat. My sense of loss from my father's death had returned. Even though it had been a year since my father died, my agony was raw and fresh. My sense of loss was enormous; I couldn't stop sobbing. It was compounded by the look of vulnerability and disappointment in my Mother's face when I left her at assisted living. It was like a kick in the gut. I was BETRAYING her. I understood her feelings, but I still believed I needed to give respite care a try. I needed help. Desperately.

As she joined an exercise class, I moved her things in from the car. The care manager stayed with her, and I continued to feel I was betraying her. At day care when I left her, it wasn't a big deal. With some Alzheimer's folks it was, but not with Miss Dixie. I noticed a couple on the third floor where the dementia patients stayed. I had seen them Saturday when Mother and I visited for a barbecue at the home. The woman seemed to be the dementia patient. Of course, in my current state of emotional disarray, I thought of my father and his concern and caregiving for my mother. Sometimes, I was sure that the stress of caring for Mother had contributed to his death. Other times I was certain that caring for her had also given him the will to live. Months later I re-examined the statistics on stress for the family caregiver and was shocked at the numbers. Mortality rates increased sixty-three percent for caregivers.[14]

*

I also thought how much I would miss my mother when she died. The pain I felt with that thought was horrendous, just awful. *My mother's care had become my purpose in life.* Later I would learn that the sorrow-filled pain I experienced was called anticipatory grief, a symptom often experienced by family caregivers.

How much my life of independence had changed in the last year! I had a sense of purpose that was almost primal. I was protective and fierce.

I approached the two-week respite care with optimism. As an only child, it was just me in this sweat equity plan for taking care of my mother. Clearly I needed some kind of back-up plan. So, assisted living respite was one possibility that I needed to test. Good old trial and error!

The day I left Miss Dixie I went back in the evening for an unannounced drop-in. My mother was in the locked Alzheimer's unit on the third floor. Lo and behold, the attendant was sitting up, but sound asleep. ASLEEP. It was seven thirty at night and she was deeply asleep.

"Excuse me," I said once, then twice. That didn't wake her up. I touched her shoulder. That DID wake her. She mumbled something about being on her break.

14.Schulz and Beach, "Caregiving as a Risk Factor for Mortality," 2215-2219.

The next morning I involuntarily transformed into my Scottish Warrior Princess persona. I raised the roof a couple of inches and the attendant, who had been working a double shift, was fired. However, there was no way to feel good about it. How good would the replacement be? The sleeping incident had also made me physically ill. As it turned out, the replacement was good and seemed to make a point of being engaged with patients, not just acting like a prison guard. Still, it was hard to feel confident about my mother's care.

My dear mother begged for me to take her and begged not to stay. The light in her eyes was gone, and her persona spoke to my betrayal of her.

"I don't want you to just leave me here," she repeated time after time. She had not noticed the sleeping attendant. I tried to explain that her stay was to be a short period of time, but of course she couldn't understand a concept like that at this point in her disease. Nor that I needed to spend time on work. "I'll help you with your work," she responded. She couldn't, of course. And she couldn't grasp that concept now. I was moving away as her protector. I was violating my part of the deal in her mind. I was overwhelmed with guilt. It was heart-wrenching.

I didn't go back to the Alzheimer's floor for two days, but I also couldn't leave her there without a drop-in follow-up. I arrived at mealtime. It had been my understanding that Mother would be taken to the main dining room for meals, so she could spend time with the less severely impaired. But there she was on the third floor sitting at a table with two severely disabled patients, "helping them eat," she said. Truthfully, I didn't see her helping them, and truthfully, their very presence depressed me.

Their heads drooped. There was no eye contact or communication. Could they be fed? Were they over-medicated to this comatose level? Or was it the disease? I wasn't sure. *This is my future,* I said to myself, but in reality it never was. The new attendant was feeding another resident whose dementia was advanced. She was attentive, kind, and patient. I was impressed.

Mother was clean and neatly dressed, but she seemed depressed. The light was gone from her eyes. I told her I had a meeting out of town, which was true, but she couldn't understand. I knew she didn't understand, but I still kept trying, no doubt to relieve my guilt.

Again she begged and again I walked away. This time I kept away until her stay was ending. The first few days of her stay had been emotionally draining for me, but by the last couple I felt good. Rested. Renewed. What I was supposed to feel!

At assisted living on Miss Dixie's last day, there I stood in her temporary room, packing up. It looked like she had picked up some new clothes. A bathrobe, nightgown, bra, slacks, blouse, and socks... This happened at home, too. If she liked something in my closet, it had a way of appearing in her closet and disappearing from mine. Sometimes that was okay, sometimes not.

The staff had told me that Miss Dixie had become best friends with another resident, Louella. I heard talking in the hallway, but all I could see was a purse. Louella's purse. Then I saw Miss Dixie. Happy. Chatting away with her new best friend.

"Oh, there she is," she told Louella when she saw me. "My daughter." *Goodness, she remembered that I was her daughter.*

As we headed home, Mother looked a little weary around the eyes and nodded off all afternoon, which was unusual. Her right leg, ankle, and foot were a little more swollen than was normal. She had convinced the caregivers to put nylon knee-high stockings on her. Another new item in her wardrobe never to be returned! I had long ago swapped out the knee-highs for stockings that were less binding. I was hoping to optimize circulation because of the skin ulcers on her feet.

When I brushed her teeth that night, her gums bled. I had urged regular brushings because of the dental care war stories I had heard about assisted living. Teeth just didn't seem to be a care priority.

In any case, Miss Dixie was happily back from assisted living. None the worse for wear.

As fall came, I found her creeping loss of judgment in daily living tasks getting to me. I was used to a routine with her care, but the unexpected dominated. She was still very mobile and would occasionally get up out of bed without my hearing her. That often meant a mess. When her night clothes were wet, she would decide to get rid of them in a completely inappropriate way. She would roam through the front part of the house and closets where I had less used clothes stored.

She pulled an evening skirt of mine out. It was in a plastic bag. And, she chose to put her smelly wet pants on my good evening skirt. A little bit correct, in that it was covered with plastic... But, risky nonetheless.

She hid stuff regularly and that made me crazy. She went through phases when she hid mail—checks that were supposed to come to me and to her. So, I had to remember to barrel to the mailbox the minute I heard the crack of metal from the mail slot from five rooms away.

She hid clothes, glasses, laundry about to be put on her bed or put away, cookies, empty cookie wrappers from day care, toilet paper folded neatly in little squares, and her stuffed animal prizes, which were her bingo winnings. Before Dad died, I could share those experiences. Now, there was no sharing partner. No wonder I missed those times.

In the fall, her glasses went missing. Funny thing was, I had been thinking we had the glasses thing down and were putting them in the same place every night. *Nice try. Didn't last long.* I had scheduled an eye examination after a four-month wait for new patients. I was sure her glasses needed to be changed, but I was uncomfortable waiting two months for a new pair. Besides, it also seemed that her hearing was worse with her glasses gone. Is that possible? So, I ordered a replacement pair from Michigan. Years later I found her glasses on the top shelf of an otherwise unused cabinet.

I had plopped a sheet I had washed on the bed. After I picked her up from day care, a business call came in. After supper I went to make her bed, and the sheet had disappeared. Disappeared. I went berserk. I stormed her usual hiding places: Dad's old closet, the guest closet, the guest bedroom, the living room, the drawers, the cabinets, the linen closet. (Silly me). I noticed again a stain from previously urine-soaked pants in the drawer of an antique cabinet. I had not gotten to that hiding place quickly enough. Nothing. Her closet. She never hid anything in there unless it was my clothes that she was reclaiming. But I thought I'd try it just in case.

If I didn't get her clothes hung in her closet quickly enough, she might fold them very neatly and stuff them under her pillow or under the covers. The Michigan house had layers of her clothes in the bedroom. We literally spent two years getting the clothes, never worn, in a variety of sizes, out of that house, and we still had bushels when I locked the door and sold it.

Her bingo creatures had been sleeping on the other side of the bed with her. Hidden sweetly beneath the covers, of course.

That sheet for her bed was a tipping point. I roared through the house twice, slamming doors to the point that I split one closet door. I finally found the missing sheet hidden under a pillow in the guest bedroom. I apologized for losing my temper before she went to bed.

"Oh," she said sweetly. She had forgotten that her daughter had been a jerk.

THE HELPING PROFESSIONS, NOT SO MUCH

The day of her eye appointment arrived. Not surprisingly, the doctor's first recommendation was cataract surgery. Both eyes, but one eye at a time with an interval of roughly four weeks before the second surgery. The doctor had a good reputation. Probably in his forties, he was an excellent technician, but with limited social skills; or at least that's how I saw him.

So, there I was, trying to process what this surgery could mean for someone who was cognitively impaired. I hadn't really thought about how I might manage a surgery before. I had been my mother's sole caregiver for about a year and a half. Colds and viruses were one thing, but surgery was unanticipated. I was fairly obsessed and overly anxious about this new wrinkle, outpatient surgery. My own information processing requires a lot of information, even when I'm not dealing with an Alzheimer's patient, so add a new caregiving situation onto that... I was close to a wreck. Not surprisingly, the doctor's staff shared his level of social skills and patient empathy, or lack thereof. I found myself in a very unsatisfactory conversation with the surgery scheduler. It was clear that she was paying no attention at all as I carefully explained my mother's fear of the dark, Alzheimer's, etc. Miss Dixie wanted everyone, including herself, home when it was dark.

"Okay," said the scheduler. "Let's have her come in at 7 a.m. on January..." *Before daybreak.* I huffed and puffed to myself. *Like talking to a stone.* "Fine," I said, knowing full well that I would cancel.

The next day I canceled the surgery with no explanation. Why try to talk with a stone? Months later in springtime, when daylight was longer, I scheduled surgery and took my little lamb to the slaughter. She had been told nothing. Yes, I finally wised up about too much information. Just another day, only a little earlier with no breakfast. She didn't notice. She was fine. I was nervous. This was an especially hard and lonely time for me, maybe because it was an unknown; a first in my caregiving. I'm not certain. Still don't know.

As I took her home, Miss Dixie was in good shape. Then, rip, rip. Off came the bandage. For two hours, I replaced the bandage and tried to convince her to leave it on. Not gonna happen. So I gave up. The next morning we checked in at the doctor's office and went on to day care. One of the folks at day care expressed some surprise that she was coming back to day care so soon. But, why not? She had medical clearance, and having activities that she was used to seemed like a good idea. After all, she had ripped the bandages off, scratched her eye continuously, and generally managed to do everything she was not supposed to do. Why not see if the distraction of activities would slow her down? Fortunately, the surgeon put an extra stitch in, so the uncontrollable behavior had minimal impact.

Meanwhile, this was not the only issue on the medical front. Skin ulcers and, later, skin cancer became issues. The ulcers started with her feet. Putting topical cream on several spots on her feet became part of our morning and evening routine. Then a minor skin problem showed up on her leg. It was a mild cancer. I kind of remember her backing into a hot steam pipe in the dry cleaners when I was a kid and getting a really miserable burn from the pipe. I figured that might have been the reason for cancer. I think I probably had a similar experience, but my burn wasn't as severe. That explained the skin cancer on her leg, but not the skin ulcers on her feet. At least two of her brothers had foot problems, so I concluded her feet might be a genetic issue.

Bedsores were treacherous in the nursing home population, but folks who were moving around were not supposed to have them. For every generalization in Alzheimer's care, there is an exception. That was my experience. *Get used to it.* Her skin ulcers were the result of poor circulation in the legs and feet, her doctor concluded. A few days before her second cataract surgery, a large, unpleasant skin ulcer made its debut on her leg. Topical cream was the treatment, but it was not healing quickly. It actually freaked out one of the nursing staff people as Miss Dixie was prepared for surgery. I guess I was getting used to it. I tried to get someone from the hospital's wound care staff to come by to look at it. Didn't work. But, I did talk with a wound nurse on the phone and was able to convince myself that I was doing an okay treatment regime, using the stuff I used for the twice-a-day wound care to her feet.

The compounding of minor events began to overwhelm me. All treatments for skin ulcers and cancer were slow to heal and took twice as long as was anticipated. The second cataract surgery was much easier, largely because my anxiety level was lower.

Miss Dixie seemed to be in stage six of the seven stages of the disease, as outlined by the Alzheimer's Association. We had occasional visits from Mother's imaginary horse. She still laughed and smiled, could walk by herself and feed herself, and said, "Thank you for helping me," as I put her to bed. Life was sometimes challenging, but manageable.

Late at Night: Working Through the Emotions

Late at night I gave myself lectures on the poor decisions I had made.

I'm alone, an only child, unmarried, childless, I celebrate aloneness, I hate aloneness, I want to be alone, I hate being alone, I want to love, I want to be loved, I don't care about love, I don't have the time or energy to care about love, I'm smart, I'm not that smart, if I had been smarter, I would have gotten better grades in college, if I had known that the choice of school mattered, I would have picked a different school, I barely made it through the school I picked, I would never have made it through a better school, I actually liked the school I picked even though it wasn't an East Coast name brand, the first people I learned to dislike in DC were name brand Ivy League types, especially lawyers, Geez, how politically dumb can you be, I came from the real world, a lowbrow land grant university and I loved the school that East Coast elites look down their respective highbrow noses at, does it hurt my feelings that elites don't think much of my school, I guess it must, but why, since I can't stand elites anyway.

What's wrong with me, it's a shame I quit drinking and smoking, I'm glad I quit drinking and smoking, and now if I could quit eating, when I get Alzheimer's I'm going to pay for being alone, I don't care, I care, I would not have been able to care for my parents if I had not been alone, very few men would have accepted both parents moving in, some men might have accepted both parents moving in, no man would have accepted both parents moving in, I had three full time jobs, working as a self-employed consultant to nonprofits, working as my father's caregiver, working as my mother's caregiver, I had no room for marriage or other family care, but who will care for me now when I get Alzheimer's, I need to die earlier than my parents did, so I probably need to die of something other than Alzheimer's, my chances of dying of pulmonary disease are improving, I think I would prefer Alzheimer's, but I may not have a choice in this, heart disease could be my cause of death too, chances are very good that my money will run out before I die anyway, and that alone could give me a heart attack, it's true that I tried to get long-term care insurance, but was turned down, and that was even before I had breast cancer or hereditary COPD, I may need to think about going to Oregon as a right-to-die state, or is it? I think so.

Alzheimer's research, why has there been so little progress in treatment or cure research with Alzheimer's, in the last thirty years it's been growing by leaps and bounds? The cynical me says, first, it's an old persons' disease, second, it's an old persons' disease, and then the big nonprofit players in the disease business have a vested interest in the status quo, otherwise why in the hell would you pay a CEO in a tax-exempt organization TWO point seven million dollars ($2.7 million) in 2012?[15] *He must have found a cure and you missed reading about it, Smarty Pants.* Not a chance.

Spitting fire won't help. It makes people mean and defensive. I know, I know, but still...

Back to the personal stuff, finding a cure is PERSONAL to me! *Yeah, but...* why didn't I have kids, it's really not that complicated, since I didn't get married and I had this notion of man, woman, marriage, children, in that order, as untraditional as I was, I didn't want to listen to the grief I would have to take from my parents, or snide small-town remarks, besides, how would I have gotten through school, since I had to work my way through, and my mother was taking my money to buy antique hall trees, *oh for heaven's sake, give that up, will you please,* but I wouldn't have been able to support a kid and myself and get through college more or less in one piece, since I nearly had a nervous breakdown as it was.

Eyes closed. Breathe in. Breathe out.

Back on the kid thing, as I mentioned earlier, my equipment was lousy, so I didn't really see as many options as women see today, and once the equipment folded, getting married made less and less sense, besides, I didn't stay infatuated very long, and commitment became less attractive, especially as friends began divorcing, and the only men I was

1511. Alzheimer's Disease and Related Disorders Association, Inc., "Form 990 for the Year Ended June 30, 2013," 13, http://www.alz.org/national/documents/FY13_990.pdf.

really attracted to wanted kids, so there I was, damaged goods, why run the risk with a serious long-term involvement, and no, I didn't want to adopt, because I didn't want to adopt, besides how many people did I know who had absolutely useless, messed-up, dysfunctional kids, or sick kids. Kids were another craps shoot.

Besides, babies scare me, I can never remember how they're supposed to sleep, backs or stomachs, what if I did it wrong, I forget how to hold them, too, because I don't want to hold them, someone actually brought me pictures of her child's birth a couple of months after I had a hysterectomy, I'm sure the intentions were well-meaning, so I said, "What do you want me to do with these, put them on the bulletin board?" Actually, I probably said, "What the HELL do you want me to do with these?" Oh, she was sure I wanted to share in her baby's birth. Like hell I did.

New subject: you can be anything you want to be, just work hard and your dreams will come true, what a crock that is, parents lie unbelievably to kids, or they tell them things that crush them forever, I started learning that when I was about six years old and told my mother that I wanted to be Queen of England, and she said I couldn't be, because the job ran in the family and the family wasn't ours, it was downhill ever since and I never quite got over it or made my peace with it, I always like to blame my parents for overblown aspirations, especially since I believed them until I was fifty, *you and Peter Pan. I suppose you believed in Santa Claus all that time as well.*

Breathe in. Breathe out.

*

Five or six years after I returned to Washington in the 1990s, I joined a meditation group, which gave me a process for facing emotions without hiding them away. Fortunately, that association occurred just as my mother was diagnosed with Alzheimer's and I became a long-distance caregiver. *Breathe in. Breathe out.*

Along with forgiving others, I learned self-forgiveness. I started to realize or believe that as hard as it was, maybe there were enough good things in my life to balance out the pain from some of my early decisions. I looked back on my life; my choices were non-traditional. Yet, inside I felt very traditional. There were some spectacular moments. I liked the proximity to history and newsmakers. There was a wholeness about it all in a crazy sort of way. One experience led to another.

I had always been around older people, seniors really. I had rarely been around babies and children. My sitters mostly had been women with white hair, and I really liked them. I had always wondered: Was I self-absorbed? Was that the reason I didn't have children? Was I like my mother? *Breathe in. Breathe out.*

I was really pretty good at family tasks. I enjoyed them and missed them when Miss Dixie was in skilled nursing. Maybe family caregiving in old age was what I was supposed to do? Maybe. Self-forgiveness was a wonderful thing. And, life purpose. My mother's care had become my life purpose. Helping others after she was gone might be my next step. How? I wasn't sure. But perhaps I could find a way.

Breathe in. Hold it. Breathe out. Solitude. Wholeness. Gratitude. Success.

BIG TIME TROUBLE—2006

Overall, life was fairly normal. Every now and then we would have people in for lunch on a Sunday. Walter and his wife Sophie, from my Alzheimer's group, lived in the neighborhood, so we decided to get together.

I also invited Janey Hart, who was the widow of my first Washington boss, Philip A. Hart, a US senator from Michigan. I had worked with Janey more than thirty years earlier. Skilled at using her position as "the wife of" in support of political and social issues about which she cared deeply, Janey was great fun. A practicing Catholic, she nonetheless opposed the Catholic Church's positions on birth control and women in the church and did so publicly and occasionally with a take-no-prisoners style in the sixties and seventies. I was certain Walter and Sophie would enjoy her and conversation would be lively.

Janey was wonderfully colorful at a time when Senate wives were staid to the point of being dull. Before she quit driving she sported an attention-getting bumper sticker that said, "Jesus was a liberal." On a red Thunderbird, of course. Yes, we all drove Detroit cars.

She said it prompted such strong reactions on the road that she eventually took it off. People screamed through their closed car windows and shook their fists at her. A mother of eight children, Janey was also the product of Michigan manufacturing prowess. Her father, Walter O. Briggs, Sr., was a legendary figure at Chrysler. So her politics ran counter to the expectations of her upbringing.

Mother and I went to pick Janey up at the Shoreham in Washington (in one of my ancient Hondas) and brought her to our house. I had made turkey chili, so it was very informal. Sophie, who was in the very early stages of Alzheimer's, and Walter were great conversationalists.

Janey and I started telling stories about our travels together in the 1970 campaign.

The senator was running against Lenore Romney, the mother of the 2012 Republican Presidential candidate. Janey had gotten herself arrested for praying at an anti-war gathering at the Pentagon. So, my major unspoken assignment was to see that Janey stayed out of trouble during our campaign in Michigan. We were both bored to death, but we became good friends, so that helped.

Later during the Watergate scandal, Janey would call me at the senator's office every morning after she read the paper with running commentary of what was outraging her. I told the story that Janey told me one morning—which was the best line ever—but a line that I could never report to the press.

"I never liked Nixon," Janey said. "But, I'm really concerned about what this is doing to the office of the presidency. Obviously, I didn't vote for him. But, I really didn't expect him to do this"— calculated dramatic pause—"shit on the chair." Then she stopped, waiting for my reaction. As expected, I dissolved into peals of laughter.

I repeated the story at lunch and we all laughed and laughed. Janey, Sophie and Walter and Mother. Especially Mother.

"And Barbara doesn't usually talk that way," my mother volunteered as she laughed. *Don't think I'd put too fine a point on that particular issue, but it was one of the great fun moments despite Alzheimer's.*

Later after a fall and head injury, Janey was put on Alzheimer's medications. She died in 2015 of complications from the disease. Alzheimer's is not very selective about its victims, the notable and less notable in it together.

*

It was raining heavily. It wasn't a hurricane, but one low-pressure system after another had settled over the East Coast in June 2006. There had been significant rainfall for more than a week. Several inches of rain had fallen each day. The ground was saturated to the point of squishing when you walked on it. My new lavender plants along the side of the house had drowned already.

I wished I hadn't been so distracted with Mother's urinary tract infection. I should have followed up when my yard service didn't show up to clean the gutters. Oh well, next week...

It was Sunday and Mother was very sick. Sleeping. Not interested in eating. Mother always loved to eat. The phone rang. The doctor's office called to say the lab reports were in on Mother's infection and the antibiotics needed to change. Once before we had to change when the cultures came in. That certainly explained why she wasn't getting better.

Since she was sound asleep, I could certainly slip out for her new prescription. Sometimes I felt guilty when I dashed to the grocery store on Sunday morning and left her in bed sleeping. I don't know why, but I did. But, not now. Let's get her started on this new antibiotic.

Later, the weather people were talking about small-stream flooding. It seemed like a lot of water, but it wasn't too scary since wind wouldn't be a big factor. Several inches of rain per hour should be expected, the forecasters said. Perhaps, fourteen inches of rain in a twenty-four hour period. *Let me revise my scary assessment.*

It was dark and overcast. The rain was heavy, really pounding. When I turned the outside light on, I could see the water pouring over the gutters all along the porch. The water was running nowhere. It was standing. I had checked the French drain. I ran to the other part of the house, the old part, to make sure there was no debris blocking the drain at the side entrance. All of the gutters were over capacity. Water was gushing everywhere. The weather people kept talking about the exceptional amount of rain.

It looked to me as though the water along the side of the house might be rising. I needed to keep an eye on the levels. It was at least eighteen inches from the door. Seemed to be a nice slope. Should hold.

An hour later another burst of pouring, pounding rain. Flipped the lights on. Water level was only six inches from the door. In a matter of minutes, water was oozing under the door and spreading on the wood floor.

Mother was sleeping soundly, but should I evacuate? I called the fire department and explained my dilemma. I needed someone to help me decide how bad this thing was going to get and should I leave? In a few minutes, the fire department arrived.

Three big hulking guys in foul weather gear came walking through the old part of the house with its twenty-eight inch doorways. The lead fireman walked through Mother's room, saw her sleeping, and I could almost see the light bulb go off in his head.

"You know. I would stay here," he said. "If you could get someone with a pump and a hose, you could run the water down the driveway." *Think, Barbara, think.*

The Timster. He was a walking, talking hardware store. An engineer. Mr. Fix-It. If anyone might have a solution, it would be the Timster. Tim Carmody was married to a long-time friend from St Louis, Joann Piccolo Carmody. Maybe Jack could help too. *Yes, Barbara, this was a full-fledged crisis. Time to call up the National Guard.*

Both men arrived with equipment, good backs, and good humor. Tim had loaned out the pump that would do the trick, but he went to recover it, and he had a hose that would send the water down the driveway. While I bailed water on the inside, Tim and Jack hooked up a pump and hose that sent the water down the driveway. Tim showed me how to work the pump and set this little engineering marvel up. Jack Cornman, a long-time friend from my Hart office days and one of my current business partners, said, "You know... you've got a lot of roof line here. It could just be the clogged eaves that are the problem." And so it was.

My mother got better. My engineered wood floor was ruined and replaced by a tile floor. Just saying it sounds so simple. However, it took months of upheaval and money. The existing wood floor and liner had to be ripped out. Thankfully, the husband of a work colleague brought a crew in and took care of the demolition in a day. While mother was in day care. Renovations around an Alzheimer's patient are not an easy thing. Again, I probably lost a couple years off my own life span during the three and a half months of renovation work. But, eventually we had a tile floor that could take water if it ever happened again. It didn't.

I learned to get the eaves cleaned when there was a whisper, a soft, faint whisper of heavy rain. Chances were it was a combination of both clogged eaves and a drainage system that for fourteen inches of rain in a twenty-four hour period needed to be more robust than a French drain. Expensive lesson, and how often did we get that much rain?

In partial defense of myself, the IRS flooded. So did the Commerce Building, the National Archives, and the Justice Department building. Roads and underpasses flooded; a century old tree on the White House lawn collapsed despite the absence of extreme wind. So, the weather conditions were challenging even for people who didn't forget to clean their gutters while caring for an Alzheimer's patient.

Oh well.

*

The world's greatest Alzheimer's support group gathered at our meeting place in Arlington in August 2006. It was the usual gang of folks except our fearless leader, Walter, was not there. It was a little unusual, but we really didn't think too much about it. There were three leaders, and we figured signals had gotten crossed.

Walter, one of the leaders, and his wife Sophie, who was the Alzheimer's patient, lived in my neighborhood just a few blocks from me. It was a second marriage and they both described the other as their soul mate. A former engineer, Walter was known about town for his volunteer work. He had won awards for it, including teaching math to prisoners in the county jail. Terrific guy. Smart. Salt-of-the-earth human being.

Sophie was equally terrific. She had been a nurse and had set up nursing scholarships early so that she could meet the recipients of her generosity. Her original intention was to make the gift in her will. Both Walter and Sophie had children from their first marriages. Walter worried openly about Sophie's children and their ability and commitment to Sophie's care. Her relationship with her son was close; her daughter seemed to be, well, a little immature. This was from Walter's perspective. That's the kind of stuff we talked about in group. Family relationships, support for the patient, support for the caregiver. But, thank heavens Sophie had Walter to look after her wellbeing as Alzheimer's progressed.

But the group. The great thing about our group was that it was filled with self-starters, so we went ahead and had our meeting as usual.

I was the keeper of the "list" so I decided to call Walter's house when I got home. A pleasant voice answered the phone.

"Sophie?" I asked.

"No, she's not here right now," came the reply.

So, I started to explain Walter's absence at group. The voice on the phone was quiet. Then, she spoke.

Walter had died on Saturday. Dropped dead on his exercise bike. He was DEAD. That's why he wasn't there to lead group.

*

In the fall, I took Mother to her routine appointment with her neurologist. Without saying much (he typed rather than talked), the doc announced that he was taking Mother off Aricept. *You're kidding,* I said to myself. *Maybe we could talk about this?* Another know-it-all physician.

It seemed that he had seen something on a heart test that he didn't like, plus "she has a history of fainting." *Really*? thought I. It has not been proven that she fainted. It was just a wild guess that that could be what happened. So, maybe we could have a conversation? Since I'm busting my ass taking care of her, maybe I could be involved in this decision. Read my lips: *I have medical and durable power of attorney. So, a consultation IS in order.*

Of course, I didn't say any of this to him, but I should have. Six months later, he was gone to Seattle and I fired the whole damn practice. But, I'm getting ahead of my story again.

Dixie and Barbara—2007

I told Mother she had a birthday coming on January 14. "You'll be ninety years old."

"Wow," she said. So, I started to make plans. Why not make this a special time to celebrate! She might not know when January 14th was, but she still knew a festive celebration from an ordinary day. Her birthday was on a Sunday, so we could have the party on her actual birthday.

It was funny how the party energized me and sharpened my focus almost to the point of obsession. Besides, I had wanted to have a party, a sort of welcome party when Mother and Dad arrived in Virginia, but Dad's health had been too precarious.

I cooked and froze during the Christmas holiday and invited old friends and new friends from my Alzheimer's support group. One person from the group brought the patient, her husband. He was very bright, loquacious, in the early stages of the disease, and had a good time. No one knew he had Alzheimer's.

Cards came in from out-of-town friends and family. I taped the cards to a ribbon that draped the window frames. Very festive. Lots of fun.

When I asked Mother's sitter to come, she said she would keep Mother entertained while I played hostess. That she did and beautifully. Miss Dixie knew the fuss was about her. She saw balloons, flowers, a fancy cake, and lots of people wishing her well. We had about twenty-five people in and out that afternoon, and a couple of people were invited after her birthday for leftovers. There was curried butternut squash soup, vegetables, fruits, curried lentils, and on and on. Yeah, I got carried away. I always figured that was all right, since you never knew how many birthdays were left.

I developed a fun plan for my own birthdays, too, since I no longer had a family member who knew when I was born. Rather than mope around, I decided to make "Happy Birthday, Barbara" signs and put them around the house. Since my mother could still read, I received her congratulations several times during my special day.

It went something like this.

Miss Dixie: "Is it *your birthday* today?"

Barbara: "Why, yes, it is."

Miss Dixie: "Well happy birthday."

Barbara: "Thank you so much." And over and over. Everyone was happy.

*

One of my truly dumb moments occurred in February. After supper I went looking for Mother. I was doing something in the kitchen but couldn't figure out where she was.

I found her slumped over sitting on the toilet seat cover. I tried to rouse her but nothing worked. Somehow... I still don't know how... I got her into the portable wheelchair and transferred to a large lounge chair—something she used to sleep in in Michigan. In my state of angst, I had lifted the lounger up and put it in the bathroom. Why? I knew I couldn't get her beyond the bathroom to her bed. I gave her sips of water periodically and continued to try to wake her.

Why didn't I call EMS? I'm not sure now. Adrenalin was pumping, but clearly good judgment was lacking. What was going on in my own thought processes at the time? Maybe I was getting self-conscious about calling EMS too often. What's too often with an Alzheimer's patient and a sole caregiver? I SHOULD be able to do this by myself. *I should*, I told myself unrealistically.

Several times when I had found her asleep in the closet, we had gone to the emergency room (ER), sat there for six hours, only to be discharged and sent home with no diagnosis. Maybe my reluctance was coming from a story I had heard in my support group? The patient fainted every now and then. None of the medical folks could figure out why. It just happened. So that caregiver had decided to stop sending the patient to the hospital when fainting happened. Bring her to and stay with her. Who knows what I was thinking!

Anyway. I called the doctor the next morning when nothing had changed. I reported the symptoms to her and the doctor's response was one word: HOSPITAL.

So, Miss Dixie was diagnosed with dehydration, the beginning of kidney failure, and probably an impacted bowel. She stayed in the hospital at least five days. The new wing of the hospital was open now with a soothing color palate and comfortable sofa beds in each room. Wonderful improvement. Much appreciated. I could work on my laptop in Mother's room with relative comfort.

During those few days, Mother forgot how to walk. The doctor said she couldn't go home safely and ordered physical therapy in a skilled nursing center to teach her to walk again. I'm fuzzy now on a lot of the details, but I remember a horrendous ice storm and a strategic planning meeting with my consulting client. Since Mother was in the hospital, I could attend the meetings. Conversations about Mother's move to a skilled nursing facility moved quickly with the social worker at the hospital. Because of the weather, I was unable to do an eyes-on inspection of the site recommended by the social worker. Big mistake!

The day of Miss Dixie's discharge came. Let's call the skilled nursing/ rehab facility "Pittville." First, we waited hours for discharge papers or an ambulance. I don't remember what the problem was at this point. The social worker told me I would have roughly $150 to pay by check to transport Mother. So, I had to hang around. At the time, it seemed a little goofy since there was no way I could get Miss Dixie into a car for the two-and-a-half-mile trip. I pushed a little for a reason for the fees, but not a lot. Here seemed to be another case of a stupid rule holding fast.

WHEN SKILLED NURSING IS A MISNOMER

Folks took Miss Dixie to the ambulance area, and I headed off to Pittville so that I could meet the ambulance and pay the drivers. Darkness had set in by the time I arrived. The first floor of the place was attractive, the second floor less so. The sounds were disturbing cries of discomfort and disability. Dirty laundry and meal trays crowded the hallways. There was a smell of discomfort and illness, not yet a stench, but a smell. I was increasingly distressed by what I saw. Besides, the energy in the place did not feel good, and there was no eye contact from the staff. I felt my stomach churn.

The ambulance driver told me that Medicare should pick up the full charge since Miss Dixie had two medical issues, Alzheimer's and degenerative back disease. So, no check was needed. I was grateful for his help. It certainly made sense since there was no way I could have transported her. Shouldn't the social worker have figured that out? *Well, yes.*

At Pittville, my mother's bed had been lowered to the floor. Apparently Pittville's interpretation of a state law or regulation was behind that decision. Restraints were not permitted in skilled nursing. Good intentions. But there was something terribly distressing about seeing my mother put on the floor to prevent her from falling out of bed. That visual image conjured up straw mats in Third World countries in my head. Then, too, there was the notion that degenerative back disease probably made her pretty much immobile at that point. So was this really necessary? Doubt it. Pittville stopped the floor placement after that first night. Perhaps, someone read her chart. Or not.

She was lifted from the gurney by a mechanical lift. So, there she was swinging through the air and about to be lowered to the floor. It felt like no one wanted to touch her. It was all creepy and unnerving. After she was settled in, I left her and returned the next day at lunchtime. Good thing I did, too. There was no one to help her eat, and she surely needed feeding assistance. Her bed was raised.

Her lips were dry and visibly parched. Where was the water with her meal? No water. Why? She had tipped over the flimsy paper cup of water earlier in the morning, inconveniencing the staff. So Pittville's solution was to pull her water. Help from an aide would cost money. Steam was beginning to come out of my ears and fire from my mouth. Much later, I learned that what she really needed was a nice crystal glass. Give her cheap, paper utensils and she spilled it. Fortunately, I had brought a sixteen-ounce bottle of water and she drank it all. Home I went to write a little love note to the administrators with a copy taped to her bed. Hydration and dental care were my two main issues, but I threw in a couple of others also.

Each time I visited I faxed another love note to the administrator, since nothing had changed with regard to her care. She would not have been able to eat had I not been there to help, either. The staff all appeared to be low-paid recent immigrants with very limited English. How much English could they read? Who knows! Further, they did not appear to have much training or commitment to patients, otherwise the sorrowful groans and cries from rooms on the corridor might have been diminished a little.

The next day I had the privilege of meeting Pittville's version of Nurse Ratched—the miserable character from *One Flew Over the Cuckoo's Nest*. Apparently my love notes were attracting attention. Of course, I continued the love notes since hydration and dental care were still issues—Nurse Ratched or not. We were polite, though testy. Nurse Ratched didn't like me and I certainly didn't like her. *Just get your underlings to do their damn jobs*, I was thinking.

Another day passed. Imagine my surprise when I discovered a message on my answering machine saying my mother had been re-admitted to Virginia Hospital Center. No, it didn't matter whether anyone was in the house to take the call. She was still going to the hospital because of some mysterious bleeding in the bowel and/or genital area. She had only been in Pittville a couple of days, but I was pretty sure they didn't like my notes. Yes, I was concerned about my mother's condition and I had little confidence in Pittville's competency. Could Pittville have made this up to get rid of us? Possible, very possible. In any case, I was pleased to have her out of there. That gave me a little time to find a more suitable facility where nursing was at least slightly skilled.

Our first visitor and meeting in the ER was with an OB/GYN. She was a petite woman with light brown hair and an overly solicitous facial expression. It was a strange conversation. The doctor had two residents or interns in tow. The doc started by telling me the bleeding was probably terminal, advanced, undiagnosed cancer. *How's that for openers?* Fortunately, I didn't believe a word she said. Some little voice inside me warned that I was talking to a fool.

"Yes, I'm sure it's cancer and advanced," she continued. I probably scowled, since she adopted an even more empathetic facial expression. *She was lucky I didn't hiss.*

Probably trying to teach the kid docs empathy, I said to myself. The death warrant conversation continued. I waited for surgery, just a D and C, and for the report. This team didn't find anything—almost literally. Her uterus was the size of a walnut, the gynecologist reported. It was all I could do not to laugh out loud. And, the walnut was not terminal as predicted. Wonder what the kid docs learned that day? That they were assigned to a silly drama queen? Oh well. The next test was for the colon. Okay there, too.

So why was she in the hospital? The tests and exploratory surgeries reinforced my speculation that Miss Dixie had been exited from Pittsford with false symptoms. Fine by me. Let's find a new place. I had given up on the places in Arlington County, so I headed to Fairfax County. Local skilled nursing facilities were frankly a little scary, but suddenly another possibility was presented to me. The Jefferson. A bed had opened at the Jefferson.

I went to see the place and loved it. What a pleasant environment! No screams and bad smells. No hallways loaded with dirty laundry and used food trays. Real dishes and silverware. Pleasant and engaging staff who seemed happy to be there. *Yes, this would be fine.*

Miss Dixie arrived, and a detailed intake interview was scheduled. So different from Pittville.

I had explained at length and explicitly about the fact that Mother's neurologist had taken her off Aricept. Why? Because he saw something on a heart test. His decision was made without a discussion with me, her medical power of attorney and sole caregiver. I didn't like the lack of consultation, but I wasn't pushing back at that point. I simply reported the background to the Jefferson staff person, who seemed genuinely interested in the no-Aricept decision.

On Miss Dixie's second day at Jefferson, I decided to do her hair. It was getting too long and it hadn't been washed for a couple of weeks now. Sometime earlier, I had bought a dry shampoo. So, I wheeled Miss Dixie into the bathroom and turned it into a hair salon. Was there even a bathroom at Pittville? Must have been. I couldn't remember.

First, her meals were pureed and delivered to her in her bed. As she got better, she went to the dining room in a wheelchair, and I sat with her to help. Really quite pleasant. Although I had not seen her therapy sessions, her eyes were brighter and the old light was back. She was getting better. In fact, she started trying to stand in her wheelchair when she saw something that interested her. Getting rowdy.

COMPLAINING FOR CHANGE

In the meantime, I wrote a letter to the hospital social worker, complaining in strong terms about her recommendation of Pittville and the fact that she told me I would be charged for Mother's ambulance trip. Bad advice all around. Based on our experience at Pittville, I argued that no patient with advanced Alzheimer's should ever be sent there. To her credit, the social worker gave the letter to her boss and her boss called me. Their notes and my recollection of our conversation did not agree. And, I held my ground about my recommendation based on our experience. I saw no redeeming features! Period. *Do not send dementia patients there!*

*

Shedding light on the good and the bad became a secondary personal mission during the Alzheimer's journey. When I was in high school, our English teacher selected an Edna St. Vincent Millay passage to describe me. "I know. But I do not approve. And I am not resigned."[16] I didn't like it one bit, but went about my life pretty much following it without deviation. This character trait was and is not necessarily a good thing. But the other side of that is: when I'm in the zone, I really don't care. Also, I felt an obligation to try to make it a little easier for others who follow. Sometimes it wasn't possible, but it was at least worth attempting.

I considered trying to file a formal complaint with the state about Pittville. It was a convoluted process for someone dealing with a frail patient. First, the complaint needed to be made while the patient was in the facility. Otherwise, it could not be investigated. Okay, I get that part. But, let's look at the situation a little more. What about retaliation

---

16. Edna St. Vincent Millay, "Dirge Without Music" in *Collected Poems*, edited by Norma Millay (Harper & Row, 1956).

that impacts the patient? Already Pittville had the nerve not to provide my mother with water. What else would they do while I was not present to advocate for my mother? My first objective was to get my mother someplace safe. So, I left Pittville without registering a complaint that would be useful to any future patients and caregivers. I felt badly about that. Word of mouth continues to confirm that Pittville is a less than desirable place, but patients still go there. My hope is that those patients are sufficiently aware to speak for themselves. Otherwise, the place is outright scary.

This situation reminded me of an old *New Yorker* cartoon I had posted on my wall in my Senate office cubicle. As I recall, it was attributed to the Army Corps of Engineers. The caption says: "When you're up to your ass in alligators, it is sometimes difficult to remind yourself that your initial objective was to drain the swamp." There's a whole lot of that in Alzheimer's care.

*

As we approached a month in skilled nursing rehab at the Jefferson, the time came for discharge. I was grateful their care had been good. Miss Dixie would be sent home with medical equipment and orders for home physical therapy.

Truth is, I developed a love/hate relationship with Medicare equipment. I loved it when the order, placed as my mother was leaving skilled nursing, arrived on time. I started to hate it when I looked closely at what was delivered, especially the semi-electric hospital bed with mattress and rails. Not long after that order came another delivery of a mattress pressure pad with alternating pump. But, the bed was a special source of my wrath.

The mattress was a complete piece of junk. It simply was not appropriate for someone with degenerative back disease. A miserable, thin piece of foam that looked like it should be prison-issue. I immediately sent it back on the truck. I pulled a mattress from an existing bed, which was better than the piece of foam. One problem though: the mattress was a little small for the width of the bed, so I got on the Internet and ordered a decent mattress for a hospital bed. It cost $200 out of pocket to us without Medicare support. And, it was a couple of weeks before I could get delivery. In the meantime, one weekend when all of my go-to people were out of town, my mother got stuck in the space between the mattress and the side of the bed. I tried everything to move her back and around. Nothing worked... so I called 911 sheepishly and apologetically. I later learned that home health workers call 911, too, if all else fails.

This particular Medicare bed listed on Ebay for $230. Medicare paid the equipment company a rental fee. And this miserable, rotten bed cost Medicare more than $1,096 over a period of time that was more than a year. Could have been more than that, but that figure is one I can document. Then came a document saying I owned the bed. I laughed out loud. Of course, when I wanted to get rid of it, the vendor wouldn't buy it back. They would take it, but not buy it.

There was a piece of paper attached to the receipt for the equipment that promised 24-hour repair service. *Yeah, right.* The hand crank mechanism fell apart in my hand. On a weekend, of course. Naturally, Miss Dixie was still in the bed, which was fairly high off the ground. Called the handy dandy repair number. No, no help available on the weekend.

I racked my brain for Tool Guys. Who was in town this weekend? And who would be able to come to our aid with relative speed? Eventually, Jay Dunn from the Alzheimer's support group came. He patiently took the lousy bed apart and put it back together in working order. *Was I grateful! Wow!*

MEDICATIONS AND PERMISSIONS

The real saga from skilled nursing came from Aricept. Lo and behold, I got a prescription for it as part of her discharge packet. What? She had been put on Aricept at Jefferson. Interesting. Shocking. Annoying. Once again, I was not consulted. I was angry, but wait a minute. Wasn't she better? Her eyes were brighter. She seemed more engaged in her surroundings. Before, it seemed like she was headed into "zombie land." Could it be the Aricept? Maybe. Let's try this experiment a little while longer.

As noted previously, there were and are not many medication options for Alzheimer's patients. The Food and Drug Administration (FDA) had approved only four for Alzheimer's patients. One, Namenda, was for later stages of the disease, while Aricept and a couple of similar drugs could be used through all stages. When this kerfuffle on heart issues first happened, I had checked the Internet. Sure enough, there was mention of potential heart issues.

A British study seemed to be the sharpest attack, while several experts in the US discounted the research method and urged careful weighing of the pros and cons for each patient. Besides, there had long been considerable debate over whether the few authorized medications actually helped patients. How effective were they and did they stop working after several years of use? No one in my support group observed a noticeable positive impact on their patient, except me. Yes, that was only an anecdotal observation, but there was not a lot to work with in Alzheimer's medications. There have been several drugs in the pipeline, but they failed as they moved to clinical trials. What have the major national players in Alzheimer's research been doing for the last thirty years? Much more needs to happen.

After hospitalization and rehab, I scheduled an intake evaluation with the Alzheimer's Family Day Center in Fairfax. I assumed that this would be our next step up the Alzheimer's care ladder. We had stopped by three years earlier, but instead found an Arlington County Day Care program for which payment was based on income. The choice between $70 a day and $16 was an easy one, given our family resources. In Alzheimer's circles, the Family Day Center was referred to as "Graduate School." They were experts in caring for early, middle, and late stages of the disease, while the Arlington County program could not provide the individual care required for more advanced cases. So, the next step for Miss Dixie seemed to be Graduate School.

Sure enough, Miss Dixie's limitations in the evaluation put her in their late stage. Her verbal skills were compromised and her mobility was too. She could not get out of the wheelchair without assistance. Emma, her daytime health aide, and I had been working hard with a team of physical and occupational therapists. I wasn't ready to give up yet. I thought we might be able to restore some more mobility, which would certainly make my life as a caregiver easier.

While Mother had been at Jefferson, I sort of assumed that this was the beginning of the downhill run. I actually scheduled an intake interview with a hospice provider. Folks in the support group had said it made sense to get hospice ready before you needed it, so that's what I did. I also did an intake interview with a home care provider, since I was sure I would need home help when Mother was released from Jefferson.

A Stunning Reversal

A month, six weeks, two months passed and we were still trying to build skills at home. A great team of physical and occupational therapists helped Emma and me. One week, like a bolt from wherever, Emma and I noticed a marked improvement. Miss Dixie could get out of a chair by herself and walk with a walker. It was pretty astounding. I knew the nurse at Miss Dixie's early stage Arlington County day care program well enough to explain what we were seeing and ask her to come to the house for an evaluation. To put this in context, Alzheimer's is a progressive disease. That means the only direction one can reasonably expect is downhill. And, Miss Dixie seemed to be IMPROVING.

Miss Dixie passed the day care entry test. She would be able to return to her first day care program. Graduate School could wait a little longer. Once again, the universe had responded to my need for assistance, and we were given six months of grace from worrisome financial burdens that would make our journey more difficult.

An Alzheimer's patient had defied the progression of the disease with the help of her medication and focused physical therapy. Miss Dixie was back. She had moved from late stage to mid-stage. For how long? We didn't know.

*

While all of this was going on, a skin cancer spot made an appearance on Miss Dixie's nose, perhaps to assure that we did not grow over-confident. So, we got the spot taken care of before she returned to the Arlington day care program. Her dermatologist sent her to a specialist for an advanced, and probably fairly expensive, procedure. The specialist, to his credit, spoke with me ahead of time, questioning the advisability of the advanced procedure. He suggested that the recommended procedure was not appropriate. Why? Her diagnosis of Alzheimer's and her age. A less advanced procedure would give her at least five years cancer-free. Even though I was beginning to think she might outlive me, I respected his intervention. The newspapers were full of stories about expensive procedures paid for by Medicare within the last months of a patient's life. This guy had the right idea. I certainly didn't want Medicare or our gap insurance paying for unnecessary procedures. *Why didn't the first doctor make this connection? Who knows!*

*

The Aricept issue was still unresolved, and we needed a new prescription. No immediate choice but to return to our first neurological practice. I had had a number of unsatisfactory communications with the doctor's office. Silly conversations. The officious chick at the front desk told me my mother had fainted. *Funny, I never saw her faint.*

So, I gathered Miss Dixie's records from the neurologist's office and prepared for a second opinion. *What a difference.* No officious desk chicks. On our first visit, the highly regarded former chair of the unit just happened to be strolling through. He asked if we were new and welcomed us. "We'll fix you right up," he said.

Not long after our trip to our new neurologist, I answered a phone call from the old neurology practice reminding us it was time for an appointment. I hoped she heard the glee in my voice when I reported, "No longer necessary!" So, I had fired the first neurology practice. Shame on them for not involving me in the decision-making process! I had learned another important lesson.

ANTIPSYCHOTIC MEDICATIONS, YES OR NO

Despite the wonderful gift of more time in Miss Dixie's first day care program, the disease was still progressing. Aggressive behavior was an issue. Two months after her return to day care, we were headed to Georgetown for an additional prescription for "happy pills," as one of the activities staff members put it.

Happy pills were really antipsychotic medications—aripiprazole (Abilify), olanzapine (Zyprexa), quetiapine (Seroquel), and risperidone (Risperdal), generally. Nothing "happy" about them, since they come with a dreaded black box warning. The black box says something like, "when used with older people who have dementia, it increases mortality." Kind of a drop-dead notice. *The wording pretty much gets your attention.*

The day care nurse was suggesting Risperdal for Mother. After our good fortune of returning to day care, I didn't want Miss Dixie to get thrown out for being a non-compliant patient. But, I also plainly didn't like the idea of antipsychotic medications. Miss Dixie had been taking Depakote and the generic valporic acid for behavior. Clearly it was not as effective as she needed. Also, it was another controversial medication. The Food and Drug Administration (FDA) had approved Depakote as an anti-seizure medication, but it was used off-label with Alzheimer's patients. Nonetheless, it did seem to help.

As I worked my way through this issue, I came to believe that the black box wording made it seem much worse than the numbers in the studies indicated it to be. I had saved an article from 2005, which was when Miss Dixie's behavior first took an aggressive turn; she kicked someone in day care.

Anyway, this study reported a mortality rate of 3.5 percent compared to 2.3 percent in the placebo group.[17] Didn't seem like an extremely high risk to me. Once again, though, research had provided very little progress on medications for Alzheimer's disease, family caregivers simply did not have much to work with. The FDA said antipsychotics were not recommended for dementia-related psychosis. The trouble was nothing else was recommended either. *Not a good situation.* It struck me as a strange irony, this lowering the death rate for a terminal disease. Was it a premise for a dark comedy, which no one should explore because of the devastating nature of Alzheimer's?

*

Otherwise, our household was rolling along. Every now and then, late at night, I would marvel at how I became a family caregiver. Unmarried, no children, and no clear history of a "nurturing personality." Taking the emotion out of the equation, I approached it as an unwritten business contract. The contract was with my father. But years before Alzheimer's, my mother had fretted about how she might not be able to make it if something happened to my father. Even though she had worked hard in the dry cleaners, my dad had not paid her benefits. So, she did not have her own social security contributions; she was the wife of... A short-sighted solution, but most of the time they were scrambling to make ends meet. So, I understood. I had told my mother that I would help her if it became an issue. Little did I expect Alzheimer's as a part of the deal.

But when Alzheimer's arrived, I committed to a kind of sweat equity caregiving plan. There were days and times when I felt overwhelmed by the responsibility. I wished there had been enough money for more "non-me" caregiving. Then again, my parents and I did have skills— life skills, creative energy, and a tenacious focus. One of the things I had always wondered about myself was: Might I have a nurturing personality? A secret side of me? I had wanted to have kids, but never moved seriously in that direction. There were reasons and excuses that that didn't happen. Some days I regretted that decision. Other days, I was grateful for it. Unresolved ambivalence.

The other thing that probably saved my sanity was that I enjoyed making fun of people. As I recalled, good girls/nice people weren't supposed to do that. Miss Goodie left my persona years earlier. My

---

17. "Quick Study: A weekly digest of new research on major health topics," *Washington Post*, November 1, 2005, HE06. Based on an abstract from the *Journal of the American Medical Association*, October 19, 2005.

humor was sometimes pointed and unkind, but humor was that way. Fortunately, I didn't have much of an audience, so I was not burdened by the need for politically correct filters. At the time things happened, I could be explosive and intense. But, after the fact, I could almost always see the humor.

Take Miss Dixie's horse—the mythological one that showed up periodically. Although I went through an earnest/righteous period in my twenties and thirties, I always loved pretend and was able to enjoy the arrival of my mother's horse. Usually a couple of times a year.

Then there was the time she flooded three rooms—her bathroom, the utility room, and my bathroom. In the brief time it took me to drag the trash cans out to the curb for pick-up, Miss Dixie managed to flood one whole corridor. Water was everywhere, with the sink hose flapping through the air. "What happened?" I asked.

"She did it," I was told. "Just happened." The mythological SHE had appeared once again. So, the real life ME ran the wet vacuum. Crawled on the floor and mopped up with old towels. Then, not right away on this one, laughed at the loopy-ness of it all. *Might as well.*

*

Not to be outdone by my mother, I was beginning to have health issues myself. The worst was a dreadful limp. I had X-rays of my back, of my knee, but nothing could be identified as a cause. The tasks of getting Miss Dixie out of bed, into the shower, dressed, and into the car were painful. Miserable. Challenging if you're healthy, those tasks were plainly dreadful with limited mobility. I used a cane and was exhausted from the chronic pain associated with any and all movement. Even my sleep was disrupted. Got up in the middle of the night. Fished through the freezer. Oh, here they are. Frozen peas. For the ache just above my knee. Twenty minutes on, back to the freezer. Try to get back to sleep.

It was a pre-existing condition, so I couldn't switch insurance. I had to stay with my marginally competent health maintenance organization. My "crack healthcare provider," as I frequently referred to it in those days, was able to identify a bad gallbladder after three or four trips over several months, but no luck with the limp and the pain. Month after month. Yeah, I read the brochures about back pain, too. I knew I was being ignored. My rage at their incompetence was simmering just below the surface. Every time I went in to the doctor, I knew it was waste of my time.

Despite my rage, I was still trying to be a compliant patient and listened when I was told to have gall bladder surgery. For two weeks, I would not be permitted to lift. Since I was anxious about my ongoing physical limitations anyway, I brought in a live-in health aide for two weeks. I felt free to rest while someone else looked after Miss Dixie.

However, Miss Dixie did decide to run away during this period of time. Happily she was found seated on the passenger side of the car. *Ready to roll!*

TRYING TO CHANGE THE DANCE—2008

There I sat in the Neurology Department at Georgetown University Hospital in Washington on a cold, miserable January day. The banner proclaimed a superior rating by patients. I knew it was true. I had felt the positive energy from the moment I walked onto the floor five months ago.

"That flower is pretty," my mother said for the third time in fifteen minutes, nodding toward the white poinsettia. I agreed for the third time in fifteen minutes.

I had finally sucked it up and fired the neurology group that had been treating my mother and annoying the daylights out of me for roughly a year. When I arrived at Georgetown, I knew I made the right decision. One of the posters on the wall touted treating the "whole person."

It had been a busy day and I couldn't help but think about it. Mother had started at a new day care program—the Alzheimer's Family Day Center. Her Alzheimer's symptoms had finally outgrown the Arlington County day care program. She had been admitted to Graduate School at the third, most advanced stage.

When I picked Miss Dixie up that afternoon, the nurse who was clinical director and the key person in the admissions process told me Miss Dixie was qualified for the second stage. She expressed surprise at Miss Dixie's functioning. When she had evaluated her eight months earlier, she tested at their stage three.

I was both delighted and annoyed at the conversation. Delighted because Mother could enter at the second stage, which had more openings. The third stage was available only two days a week. Annoyed because I had been asking Ms. Nurse to re-evaluate Miss Dixie for six weeks. *No response. Nothing. Like talking to another healthcare stone.*

Since I was still working, I had to hire a home aide for the other three days. I even asked the nurse from Mother's first day care program to email her colleague, asking for an evaluation of mother's status in an attempt to encourage a new evaluation. Still no response. If Miss Dixie had been evaluated, Ms. Nurse would have seen that Miss Dixie did not need to be restricted to the advanced care stage. It would have save me all kinds of busy work.

I couldn't afford to go through an agency for a home health aide, so I got a tax number to pay the appropriate taxes for my "new" employee. I advertised and interviewed possible candidates and on and on. All for nothing, of course. Because someone refused to do her job in a timely fashion. It took me two years to stop the scolding notices from the Commonwealth of Virginia on my "failure" to pay taxes on my non-existent employee. Really aggravating.

I decided not to address this issue with the executive director, since I didn't want to start off with a complaint. After all, this nurse seemed better than the previous one who had interviewed us four years earlier. Still, I was annoyed that someone who was supposed to help family members had instead contributed to lots of extra caregiving work for me. I wanted to scream: "You're supposed to help me, not mess with me." But, I didn't.

Impatient, prickly me. All of this happened while I limped badly and was trying to sort out the incompetence of my health care provider. It was a character flaw on my part, I knew. Incompetence makes me crazy. People who refuse to consider new information also make me crazy.

Interestingly, this nurse was terminated a few months later. Then I explained my experience and distress to the executive director to help assure her that her decision was undoubtedly appropriate. Oddly, I was still glad that I had not complained. The center was still a wonderful place and I was especially grateful for the energy and joy that the staff conveyed.

Miss Dixie was indeed an anomaly, the anecdotal exception. She had a progressive disease but the progression had been stopped by a medication that is increasingly judged to be ineffective.[18]

---

18. "Alzheimer's drugs cost a lot, but help just a little," Consumer Reports, December 2012, http://www.consumerreports.org/cro/2012/12/alzheimer-s-drugs-cost-a-lot-but-help-just-a-little/index.htm. In 2008, the American College of Physicians and the American Academy of Family Physicians reached similar conclusions.

I had some trouble adjusting to Miss Dixie's new day care program for other reasons, too. I had grown used to the space of the Arlington Madison Center. It was a big, old school house re-purposed as an adult day care center with recreation classes for the general population. The new quarters, though more attractive in many ways, seemed more crowded to my claustrophobic self.

But Miss Dixie didn't miss a beat, literally. When I arrived to pick her up a little early because it was her first day, she was clapping her hands to the music and completely engrossed. She wasn't ready to leave, so I enjoyed the music with her a little while.

"Does your mother have a musical background?" the nurse asked. "No way," I replied. My dad had been the musical one. My mother didn't even sing along with the congregation in church. She was musically very self-conscious. Her self-consciousness seemed to be released by Alzheimer's. I had expected her artistic side to be reflected in painting and visual art activities, but it wasn't. Music was a new strong interest with Alzheimer's, and she had no previous history of interest.

Despite the blip in our start at the center, it was a wonderful place. The babble coming from Alzheimer's patients is often excruciating. It's fine to say it's just the disease talking, but how hard it is to take that pounding hour after hour.

One day when I was visiting, I heard a patient say, "You're fat." Over and over. One very capable staff person was pregnant and it seemed that I could see pain in her eyes as she heard this nonstop abuse. How tiring and difficult. All day long! "You're fat. You're fat. You're fat."

*

Despite Miss Dixie's ability to participate with others in music activities, there were other signs that her disease was progressing.

At the ophthalmologist's office, we settled in with the technician and office manager who did the preliminary testing for vision. I mentioned that Mother, at ninety-two, had stopped reading recently and therefore might not be able to read the eye chart.

"Why was that?" she asked. "She has dementia/Alzheimer's," I reminded her.

Sure enough, Mother thought the E looked like a 3. "No, not a number, a letter," the technician said, speaking complete nonsense to an Alzheimer's patient with growing irritation in her voice. I was fascinated that an E could look like a 3 to Miss Dixie. Flip it over and it could make some sense. I was actually impressed and curious about what her brain was telling her, but not the technician.

In fact, she was beginning to freak out. "She could read in July," the tech said to me. "Yes," I agreed. I wanted to growl back, *"That's why dementia is considered a progressive disease. Things change."*

Another adventure with a Medical Dumbledore. In the meantime, Mother was urging me to cheat and tell her what the letter was. I could see her mouth the words, "Help me."

Now, I ask you: who was the smartest person in the room that day?

*

My friend and hairdresser, Roi Barnard, noticed a fascinating article in *Newsweek* about "pleasant dementia" and brought my attention to it.[19]

My stories about my mother reminded him of "pleasant dementia." I have to say it reminded me also. It doesn't show up a lot in the literature about Alzheimer's since it appears to be a small subset. In my mother's case, it also was replaced in later stages by a violence that could be stunning. Fire in her eyes, rage across her face. I had to learn to leave the room to change the energy. Most often it happened when I was trying to get her moving in the morning because of my work schedule or needs. If I left the room for five minutes even, took deep breaths and repeated a meditation mantra—I could sometimes return to the room with the energy changed. But, I'm getting ahead of my story again.

The Alzheimer's decline that I experienced and that many in my support group experienced was plateau-like for a long period of time, perhaps months. Then, there was a drop where functional skills like reading changed. Sometimes I could feel the approach of a decline. Small things pointed to a lower plateau, a greater loss of functional capacity. Milestones like birthdays were especially painful for caregivers because it often highlighted where the patient was at the last birthday. That was one reason why I chose to celebrate and enjoy birthdays. The distraction

19. Sara Davidson, "My Mother's Case of Pleasant Dementia," *Newsweek*, September 9, 2008.

was useful for me, as well as entertaining for Miss Dixie.

LUCKY TRIPLE EIGHT

It was a steamy hot day. August 8, 2008. Lucky Triple Eight in China. The parking lot was so full that I parked in the sun on the rooftop of my dreaded health maintenance organization (HMO). A little early for my follow-up with the surgeon on my biopsy. *Eyes closed. Deep breaths. One, two, three. Meditate for a moment.* In that brief time, I knew I had been wrong. Wrong for six months. I assumed that I did not have breast cancer. I assumed. Now, I knew my thinking was wishful. That's all. I had breast cancer. *What was ahead for me? How would I care for myself and my mother? I was an only and alone.*

*

The top rule of caregiving was **take care of YOURSELF first**. Made sense and it shouldn't be that hard, I believed. Years ago, when I blurted out, "Come live with me," it never occurred to me that my own health might crumble. I was a member of the Silent Generation. I played by the rules; I was responsible, careful, and systematic. I was self-employed, had health insurance, and didn't run to the emergency room for routine primary care. I belonged to an HMO. It was supposed to be good; if not good, certainly adequate. I paid $800 a month for health care that was all inclusive, including flu shots and prescription services, usually with modest co-pays. I was careful to get physicals on time and took my blood pressure medication regularly. On and on. As long as I had no significant health issues, it worked well. But when I needed medical skill and treatment—it was a disaster. More significantly, it was torture that seemed to be delivered by a level of incompetence bordering on sadistic. No one could be that damn dumb. Or could they?

Why is health care important for caregivers? It goes beyond the obvious. A landmark study in 1999 reported a sixty-three percent mortality rate increase for stressed Alzheimer's family caregivers when compared to a non-caregiving control group.[20] The window of concern was four years. I assumed that most of those caregivers were of the same generation. But, after my own experience, I didn't assume anything. My problem was finding competent diagnostic and clinical care within the HMO, and I was trapped in the HMO because I had conditions that other insurers would have called pre-existing.

As a further incentive, my grandmother's Alzheimer's caregiver, Lucille, failed to keep up with routine physicals and died two years after my grandmother. Two years. Her death occurred from leukemia. It likely resulted from treatment for an advanced cancer that she had fought for several years while caring for my grandparents and still teaching. So often with hands-on caregivers, their responsibilities serve to encourage putting off basic screenings for themselves. It became a risk worth taking from the caregiver's perspective, as a result of too much to do.

Because of my Aunt Lucille's experience, I knew absolutely that I had to tend to my own health. But I couldn't get my healthcare provider on the same page. The details were so ludicrous that my HMO was like a clown act. Not quite a Third World health delivery system, but close. Their Keystone Cops antics pretended to do health care. Arrogance and ego accompanied the incompetence most of the time. In fact, I created an email list to share details and my caustic observations, which got me cheerful and much-needed feedback. Fortunately for readers here, though, my computer crashed and I lost all of my deliciously biting commentary.

*

Competence was the big issue. My primary care physician was Dr. R. She and a number of other HMO doctors displayed marginally proficient skill when attempting to provide for my health. Dr. R and I were of the same generation. We both had hair that was streaked with gray; her hair was parted in the middle and long, past her shoulders. She looked fit and trim; I did not. We were roughly the same height.

For five or six appointments, she walked in and introduced herself. Quietly, I muttered, "Yes, I know." In one appointment when I was limping, she urged me to consider wearing her brand of shoes. They were ugly, looked and sounded cheap. Over the years I had learned to recognize her footsteps. Hearing that cheap clip-clopping coming down

---

20. Schulz and Beach, "Caregiving as a Risk Factor for Mortality," 2215-2219.

the hall brought a rustle of dread even before she opened the door.

For some reason, she reminded me of the doctor who did my first major GYN surgery when I was thirty. I asked him a specific question, and he replied with complete nonsense. He simply wasn't listening. I learned then that physicians could be less than perfect, and he quickly became my former doctor.

Later I worked at a medical college and hospital as a fundraiser, one of my favorite jobs actually. So, I knew physicians who were good and others who became morticians.

The HMO guy who cut my gall bladder out looked nervous at 7 a.m. on the day of surgery. That's unsettling to a patient. My gall bladder episodes started in 2003 when I was a long-distance caregiver. A couple of times I barely made to the plane. It was diagnosed in 2007.

During the roughly twelve years that I was Dr. R's patient, I'm proud to say that she learned how to type. When the HMO changed computer systems, it had been painful to watch her at the keyboard. I always suspected that she probably grew up looking down her nose at the kids who took typing. After all, she was going to medical school. So it seemed like a real comedown for her to be forced to do her own typing. Her confidence long, long ago gave way to arrogance. Typing was really a class thing for her age group, also mine, educated before Title IX. Lesser types took typing, not the professional class. Fortunately, I was a lesser type. My Mountaineer Tiger Mother insisted on typing as a necessary life and survival skill.

Once I tried to sneak away to another primary care doc, but Dr. R blocked the attempt. Later, I was afraid if I forced the issue I might get someone worse. In fact, I even asked a friend with a health administration master's degree for advice on switching docs. He said Dr. R was probably the best at my HMO location. So, as I saw it, I was weighing "not very good" against "dreadful." Basically, I didn't have the gumption to change.

While the gall bladder episode was going on, I had terrible pain in my right leg, nonstop.

"I can't walk," I kept saying. "That's what really bothers me. I have pain walking. I don't sleep. Getting my mother in and out of bed is awful. This gall bladder thing happens every now and then. But my pain walking is ALL the time."

"We've got to take care of the gall bladder," said Dr. R.

Once she suggested Bengay for my leg. Seriously.

More than misery, chronic pain eats away at energy levels and, more seriously, one's spirit. What it does to motivation and sense of self-worth is vicious. Pain was pulling me down into a vortex of disability and despair. If I managed to get some sleep, within an hour of waking up, I was exhausted. And, depressed at how hard I had to work at every movement. Most of all, I knew my body. I was absolutely certain the problem was fixable, if only I could find cooperative, competent medical care.

"Couldn't we spend time on an all-of-the-time problem?" I asked. Dr. R bobbed her head up and down while she kept typing. The head-bobbing didn't mean yes. It simply acknowledged that I was talking. She spent most of my appointment time typing, updating my record, rarely examining.

People who are able to make HMOs work spend a lot of time working the system. I did not have the inclination to do that. No, that's not quite right. Thousands of dollars a year and no health care. I was angry and annoyed. Mad as hell, actually. Why couldn't I get what I was paying for? Why? Plus, it was one goofy episode after another.

There Dr. R sat, typing away across the room while she asked questions. Never ever in this one particular appointment did she approach me on the table, or ask me to do certain movements, or, for heaven sake, touch my leg, my back, or my hip. I'm not exaggerating. I saved my emails.

> 7/16/08 9:08 PM
>
> ... I am wondering why meralgia paresthetica was a diagnosis... What symptoms did I display that pointed specifically to this diagnosis?
>
> I don't remember that you examined my leg...
>
> And, the symptoms of the condition by the National Institute of Neurological Disorders and Stroke are NOT characteristics that I display. No rush, just curious... A good diagnosis?

In other words, my symptoms don't fit. Her response:

> 7/21/08 8:16 PM
> Well, we would have to re-evaluate in the future, but I can't
> change a previous impression...

In other words, she needed a diagnosis. It didn't have to make sense!

Finally, after a year and a half of complaint, I convinced her to give me another referral to a physical medicine physician. In contrast to Dr. R, Dr. T checked in at the computer, but spent a lot of time looking at my leg. He found a muscle that he said had not moved. He also found a "strained" muscle. So, he ordered an X-ray. A doctor who listened and examined. What a concept!

*

Another time, something didn't quite check out with my mammogram. Every year for roughly the last three, I had asked about stopping hormone therapy at my annual physical. I'd been taking it forever. Finally, I looked it up. *Twenty years, twelve years as a patient of Dr. R.*

After an inconclusive sonogram, I was scheduled for a core biopsy. The biopsy played out like the Abbott and Costello routine of "Who's on First." Dr. R said Dr. Z would give me the results. Dr. Z said Dr. R would. Finally Z gave me the results. He sounded a little surprised at the report: pre-cancerous hyperplasia. Minor angst, but I decided to hold off on further invasive procedures. My life was too complicated.

Three months later I had another sonogram. There was a new doctor, Dr. C. He expressed surprise at the previous core biopsy, since the radiologist had taken a sample from the "wrong" area, and even that was pre-cancerous. No wonder Dr. Z seemed surprised. A real confidence builder. So, Dr. C was going to rectify this wrong. Plus, he said I should have a surgical biopsy, since there was clearly an issue to be concerned about there. *Okay, okay.* Chop, chop, it was.

Meanwhile, I, the patient, was becoming a raving lunatic on the matter of finding the right spot. My hair was on fire over the screw-ups, and smoke was coming out of my ears over the impact on my life as a caregiver. All of it seemed to fall on deaf ears. I absolutely wasn't interested in more procedures performed with incompetence. Dr. C told me he could fix the wrong spot problem. Yes, fix it.

Contrasting Medical Care

As I was getting ready for chop/chop, Mother got sick, of course. She was started on an antibiotic for a probable urinary tract infection. But, by Saturday I doubted whether the antibiotic was doing its job. Once again, it took a couple of days for the culture to come in from the lab, and a different antibiotic was to be ordered as a result of the culture. We had been through this before. My tumbling, shrieking anxiety gave way to one foot in front of the other. Not much time for me and my health issues. Maybe that was a good thing.

On the weekend, Miss Dixie was just not herself, and by Tuesday I was certain she was sick enough to warrant a trip to the Emergency Room. When I was unable to rouse her and get her moving, I called the Emergency Medical Service (EMS) and she went by ambulance to the hospital. She was diagnosed with a urinary tract infection—our first in about a year and a half. She was hospitalized overnight so antibiotics could be administered intravenously (IV), except she kept ripping the IV lines out.

Miss Dixie's doctor worked with my schedule. We got Mother out on Wednesday, since her doctor knew I needed a surgical biopsy on Thursday. The secret I had been keeping from the HMO was that the minute Medicare kicked in, I was out of their stinking system and going to see a doctor with competencies. It was the end of July and I turned 65 on September 2. Medicare did not limit treatment for pre-existing conditions.

Mother's doctor, who would be my new provider, took one look at me. "What's with the cane?" my new doctor asked. Followed by, "What's the surgical procedure on Thursday?" *Self, it's going to be a real treat to deal with a human being in a white coat. Meanwhile, try not to kill anyone. Scottish Warrior Princess, I'm talking to you.*

*

So, the HMO doc told me they had a way to get the right spot. It sounded like a decent plan. Numb the area and insert wires and needles to find the marker, so the surgeon could find the right spot. *Okay, let's get this over.*

NUMB THE AREA. Relax. Breathe in and out. Searing, burning pain. Something was wrong. Excruciating pain. I was reminded of an abscessed tooth before the numbing kicked in.

"I'm not numb," I said. No response. More pain. I complained again in a louder voice. Still no response. My frustration exploded. *Hit, kill the son of a bitch.* Instead, I just sobbed. LOUDLY. One after another. Finally, the stunned radiologist apologized. *Too late.* I would have none of it.

"You people are unbelievable," I said.

"You know," he said, "this area of the body is really, really sensitive." He was telling me, the patient, WHY there was pain after he screwed up the numbing. Incompetence turned to torture at that point, as I saw it.

Eventually, I was turned over for operating room preparation. A nurse in total innocence approached me with a cheery, "How did it go?"

Teeth clenched, hands raised, eyes ready to kill, I said, "Do not come near me. I have had it." Wisely, she turned on her heel and left. I had some time to gather my rage in. I needed to breathe in and out quietly before I went under the knife for the surgical biopsy.

In the background, I heard my surgeon, who I liked, on the phone with the pathology lab. She was giving them a lecture on specimen labeling. *Why did this stuff happen within earshot of me?*

Put me under and get this surgical biopsy over.

Resting at home later that day, my phone rang about 4 o'clock. The HMO's physical medicine doctor, Dr. T, called to report on the X-ray of my right hip saying he saw something DISTURBING.

"It looks like you have severe arthritis in the right hip. I'm ordering an MRI," Dr. T said.

A year and a half later. The pain could be explained. It could have been diagnosed with a routine X-ray, a simple X-ray. It was not some malingering, difficult-to-diagnose back problem. My right hip joint was

GONE. Shot. Disintegrated. Eighteen months at $800 a month; that's more than $14,000. Couldn't we have come up with this $14,000 ago?

I gave Dr. R a few points for the failed attempts—knee and back X-rays. Still, she was a poor diagnostician, and that undermined her competence as an HMO gatekeeper! Was it because she was unskilled, unsystematic, or omnipotent in her belief in herself? Or, all. I never figured that out.

VINDICATION! A horrible day in and about the operating room, but vindication after a struggle of a year and a half. I was not crazy!

*

Lucky Triple Eight again. After the surgical biopsy another surgery, a lumpectomy, was scheduled. Later, after a week of gaining energy and reducing anxiety, I was suddenly zapped again. My creative juices were worn out. When my anger went, so did my energy. I stayed relatively calm. I emailed the people I needed to email and some I didn't need to. My cancer was estrogen-sensitive.

Then, at four in the morning, I cried. I was beginning my fifth year as sole caregiver for my ninety-one-year-old mother, who had stage six out of seven stages of dementia, according to the Alzheimer's Association definitions. My last vacation was nine years ago. I felt alone, so very alone. And tired, very tired.

Mother in her morning shower had decided to amuse herself with playful hitting. I was NOT in the mood.

"Do you know what cancer is?" I asked her. "No," she replied sweetly. "Well, it can kill you," I growled. "They are going to tell me today whether I have cancer."

*

A day or so after the lumpectomy at the end of August, my mother had a major case of diarrhea. Eventually, I got her cleaned up and to bed. I crawled around on the floor with a mop, pail, and rubber gloves. Then, I stopped and had a gut-wrenching cry. I was sad, miserable, and still a little frightened. The tears kept coming. I was tired. How much more could I handle?

Next. My surgical site became infected; it was oozing fluid. After my mother was put to bed, I went to the HMO Urgent Care. It was about

11 p.m. when I checked myself in. In another hour, I would be Medicare eligible. So, there I was, having additional tests as the clock ran out.

The lab came to me, since I was limping badly by that time. I was encouraged to rest lying down in an examining room, without going out to the miserable chairs in the lobby for the hour or so that we waited for the lab results. "It's interesting," I wrote in my journal, "... I think this is the most accommodating that the HMO has been during the more than ten years that I have been with them." Too late and too much ignored agony.

*

If you were going to have breast cancer, my cancer was the one to have. Low-grade. Noninvasive. No chemo, maybe some radiation. And, Tamoxifen for five years. Almost "cancer lite." That's what it looked like on paper. What if more went wrong? I pushed that thought out of my mind.

*

In another day, I would have an appointment with my new primary care doctor, who I trusted. My blood pressure dropped twenty points in that visit. My antibiotic for the surgery site infection was changed.

"It's the wrong antibiotic for the bacteria," my new doctor said as I showed her the lab report. No surprise there. Although the sadistic ordeal with the HMO was over, I still had follow-up cancer decisions to make. Oncologists, specialists, first and second opinions. Seven weeks of weekday radiation? That was the recommendation from my HMO. Fortunately, one outside specialist gave me the information I wanted to hear: the benefit of radiation was statistically minimal in my case, and I was comfortable skipping it.

Three months later, I became the proud owner of a new metal hip. I also discovered that Vicodin made me mean. Very mean. The Scottish Warrior Princess was yelling at the world. With my new team of medical providers, I prepared for hip surgery by arranging twenty-four hour live-in care for Mother and me. I showed Mother a picture of what was going to happen. In that brief, passing instant, she understood it.

"That's gonna hurt," she told me. Yes sir, you couldn't fool Miss Dixie. She was no HMO dummy.

Lucky Triple Eight? Yes, still lucky. Cancer lite. As it turned out, it was just my turn.

Sarsaparillas, Scotches, and Sorrows

Truth be known, John M. (Jack) Cornman and I used to drink more than a sarsaparilla after work for several years. I first met Jack, though I often called him Cornman and he called me Kincaid, in US Senator Philip A. Hart's office in February 1969. (My mother called him McCormick.) That was the week Jack and Donna's third and last child was born. Technically, we in the office met the two other Cornman tykes that week also. Dad was babysitting. It was the beginning of a friendship with the Cornman family that has lasted a lifetime.

On cold winter days, the tall mahogany doors of the Old Senate Office Building would burst open. There was Jack in a Russian-Cossack-style hat. It was cold standing at the bus stop. He threw his hat on his desk, which was piled high with papers. His body language said angry, mad as hell.

"Fuck Joe Alsop," he screamed at the top of his voice. *Ah yes, the Vietnam War.*

I didn't read the editorial page in the morning. In fact, probably the most important thing I read was my horoscope. I would look up and smile pleasantly. "Good morning, Jack."

Jack and I worked together for twenty-six years, including twelve years in a limited liability partnership along with the late Roy (Rip) R. Coffin. Jack was an agnostic, leaning toward atheism, and a Democrat. Rip, probably a Republican, became an Episcopalian priest in middle age. And I was a Democrat and a theological roamer, dabbling in religious experience without underlying strings or the closing of options. It was a strong resilient partnership until...

Jack and Rip had known each other forever. Both had been raised on Philadelphia's Mainline. Though they were different class years, both had gone to Haverford School and on to Dartmouth. Rip got an MBA from the University of Michigan and came to Washington to work at the Bureau of the Budget and Department of Labor before entering the ministry in 1973. Jack went from college to bartending on St. Thomas, or something like that. Then, he wrote obituaries in St. Petersburg, FL, and I wrote obituaries in Alma and East Lansing, MI. Jack came to DC to work in politics in the heady 1960s, working first for Senator Bob Bartlett of Alaska and then Phil Hart.

Our after-work libations didn't begin until the Cornman kids were older. Whew, did we have celebrations and sorrows! Many events called for conversation and an adult beverage. Cornman and I would pause for a sarsaparilla after I moved to Arlington in 1980, when we worked together at the National Rural Center. Our celebrations were mostly connected to the Washington Redskins, who were pretty good in those days. We told someone on the subway the name of our favorite Arlington saloon, the Lamplighter, and the guy said, "Oh yeah, my mother goes there."

"Hmm," we said, "old people and us."

Scotch whiskey was three bucks, maybe even for a double. We were there in that dark red faux-leather booth, dimly lit with hurricane candles, when we heard that one of Robert Kennedy's sons was dead. Years after the assassination, a hush *still* came over the bar at the mention of the Kennedy name.

Then there was the day turning into night when Air Florida Flight 90 crashed into the Potomac. What a nightmare. The plane crash, a crippling snowstorm, and a subway crash with the system's first fatality. Gridlock. Since we couldn't get to Virginia, we started drinking in the District that night. *Very large bar bill.*

By that time, Jack had gone through the death of Senator Bartlett after heart surgery, the death of his own mother, and then the death of Phil Hart. Jack sobbed uncontrollably at Hart's final appearance before the Michigan press corps, and I sobbed uncontrollably at Hart's funeral. It was awful, but you get used to leaning on family in tough times, and we certainly learned that while the senator was ill. We were work family.

Janey Hart, the senator's widow, always said she thought the fact that so many of us stayed friends after our time in the office was "one of the distinctions of Phil's staff." There was a special bond as a result of that painful, extraordinary life experience of his illness and the need to carry on his work as best we could while the senator was dying. At first, no one dared think that the senator would NOT survive. He had decided before the cancer diagnosis that he would retire. We imagined him writing thoughtful and erudite commentary on the issues of the day, perhaps at Georgetown, and we were heart-broken when it became clear his life would be greatly shortened. It was tempting to rage about the unfairness of it all, but it was futile, too. Perhaps that was the most significant life lesson from 1976 that Jack, other long-time friends, and I learned. Mourn, but move on with life and still try to make a contribution.

Certainly Jack was one of the first to be tested. He was preparing for a board meeting at the rural center. He received a call that his older brother Jim had been killed in a horrendous car accident. Jim and wife Betty had been bringing daughter Julie home on a college break. A huge tire had flown off a massive truck and taken the top of Jim's car with it. Miraculously Julie had reached up from the back seat to turn the motor off, or the carnage would have been even more devastating. It still turns my stomach to write about it.

Then there was Jack's dad, my grandfather, my grandmother, my very special Uncle Herbert, and my Aunt Lucille. Still not the most difficult...

The Cornmans' annual Christmas tree decorating party became the point of connection as the years went on. Donna, a fabulous cook, always had gourmet food with lots of good wine. I'm sure that's where I first met Rip and Carol Coffin.

By the mid-nineties, I was once again looking for work. I wanted desperately to leave a miserable working atmosphere where I was a fundraiser for a CEO, who had no social skills with which to bond with donors and no compunction against cover-her-ass outright lying. It was Washington, and there was a lot of that going around. Truthfully, I don't mind a little lying, particularly if it's creative with some charm. But, not the case here.

Actually, she was not my most egregious CEO, either. That was probably the CEO of Allegheny Health, Education and Research Foundation (AHERF), which was the country's largest nonprofit bankruptcy—roughly $1.5 billion in the late 1990s. The CEO did a few months in jail after 1,500 criminal charges were reduced down to a single

212   Barbara K. Kincaid

misdemeanor of misusing charitable funds.[21] He pleaded "no contest" after messing with endowment funds. The alums, mostly women of the old Medical College of Pennsylvania, didn't trust him long before his fall. I was gone by the time the final unraveling occurred, but the seeds of highly aggressive expansion and the underlying fear were there already.

Jack, Rip, and I settled into forming our own business. We provided strategic planning, fundraising, and leadership transition advice to nonprofit organizations. Generally, we emphasized small groups with annual budgets less than $3 million. All three of us were analytical types. Jack had a background in aging issues. Rip had expertise in leadership transitions and had been instrumental in the founding of the Interim Ministry Network for congregations in transition, following the departure of a minister. Departures often meant turmoil. Circumstances, as Rip would put it, that called for mediation and healing before the congregation was in a sufficiently healthy position to recruit new pastoral leadership. And, I had broad experience developing fundraising programs, marketing messages, and plans consistent with the strategic mission of organizations.

I really enjoyed the business. Each of us, especially me, was willing to settle for more modest income as a trade-off for confidence in the integrity of our purposes and practices. We met once a month, often at my house in case Miss Dixie was home from school. Jack took the minutes and Rip was the accounting person. I did the newsletters and website. Only he or she who was working got paid, so we were really independent contractors coming together for moral support and advice. Some of our business meetings were entertaining, with much of the content off the record, but we really did keep records and transact business, too. For several years we had an annual lunch at Rip's club, the renowned Chevy Chase Club. I always urged that we take a photo in front of the sign at the club for our "annual report." Trouble was we didn't have an annual report.

Our work family had challenges, too. First Jack had cancer, and then Rip. Initially each did well with treatment, but there were other challenges to come. The Cornmans' forty-year-old son, Geoffrey, a successful businessman and father of two young daughters, was diagnosed with

21. Dan Fitzpatrick, "AHERF's ex-chief bitter about his fall," *Pittsburgh Post-Gazette*, November 4, 2007, http://www.post-gazette.com/business/businessnews/2007/11/04/ AHERF-s-ex-chief-bitter-about-his-fall/stories/200711040193.

brain cancer. The spot was watched. Then, symptoms pushed Geoff and his wife to pursue every treatment option. Month after month of painful decline, and once again, how could one even conceive of treatment failing in one so full of life? But, it happened. Geoff died in July 2004. Rip was there supporting in every way possible. I was less supportive since I had just moved my parents to Virginia, and my father died a month after Geoff.

I walked into the Cornman house and headed to hug Donna. "Oh Barbara," she said. "This one's a bitch."

Then, Rip and Carol learned that their daughter Cindy, the mother of two young children in Wisconsin, was diagnosed with an aggressive form of breast cancer. She and her husband Erik fought hard. I have kept Rip's journal notes since they gave me courage and perspective for my own challenges. In 2008, Rip wrote:

"Talk about denial! My scans had been clear for a year and a half and I thought Cindy was just going through a rough patch...

"Well, as we learned in January when we went to Madison (Wisconsin) to help take care of grandkids during one of Cindy's rounds of chemo, this was the home stretch for her. We spent a very cold month while she was in an excellent hospice facility for two weeks and then stayed on for a memorial service there... Back home there was another memorial service at St. Columba's..."

In that service, Rip officiated:

"At the memorial service in Madison the admiration of friends there for her gritty courage in living with her cancer stood out. She participated in a triathlon for cancer survivors the past three years—even when she had to walk instead of run and skip the bicycle leg this past summer.

"Truly, her life was a gift worth celebrating."

That was March. In May 2008, while Rip and Carol were in Chicago attending a meeting, they received the report. His cancer had returned. In July chemo started again, and after numerous difficulties, including pneumonia, he wrote:

"The bottom line is that my cancer can't be cured; with antibiotics and the insertion of a 'J' tube, pneumonia can be eradicated and nutrition can be restored. We are exploring ways in which I can enjoy eating again.

Some quality of life can be enjoyed for a time; I am not yet terminal."

At the end of August, I was dealing with my reluctant health care provider, my crack HMO. I was walking with a cane from my undiagnosed limp and enduring nonstop incompetence in procedures for breast cancer. I was at home after an outpatient lumpectomy. The telephone rang. It was Rip, my unofficial pastoral counselor, checking to see how I was despite his own health. Here was a dying man, who still made it a point to inquire about *my* health. It is impossible for me to articulate the gratitude I felt.

A few days later, on September 10, Rip died.

Months later in 2009, Jack and I dissolved the partnership. For me, I just didn't want to gather around the table for a meeting without Rip. Jack and I never spoke of it directly, but it wasn't the same. So, I retired four years earlier than I intended. My own health had become too great a challenge when combined with the care of my mother. And, I was increasingly aware of the stunning precariousness of life. Loss had become a theme personally and professionally.

HELP COMES IN DIFFERENT PACKAGES

Help comes in different packages in the Alzheimer's caregiving business. Friends, old and new. Sitters from Craigslist, which, believe it or not, was a really great source of companion-type sitters in the early days. I also sent a recruitment email to an Episcopal seminary in the area and found some wonderful sitter/companions.

As Alzheimer's advanced, cab driver John D from Red Top Cab was a terrific go-to-guy. I would take Mother to day care in the morning and John D would pick her up from day care as part of the Arlington-County-supported transportation service. It was supposed to work on a first-come, first-serve basis. But that raised too much anxiety for me. The idea of having someone different deal with my mother each day didn't make sense from my perspective. Miss Dixie was still crafty and could confuse the living daylights out of the uninitiated.

My mother, even in her deepest Alzheimer's moments, could make royal announcements.

"Take me back. I don't live here," she would order with a wave of her hand, and the poor innocent guy, often with limited English-language skills, would believe her and start to turn the car around. At moments when her royal highness was doing her thing, she seemed perfectly rational. Her ability to bamboozle remained impressive.

Having the same guy over and over meant she couldn't fool him. So as the trip tickets were handed out each morning, John made sure he got Mother's.

Besides, she liked John D. I always figured he reminded her of her brothers. Tall and approachable, he would walk into day care and ask, "Is there someone here named 'Dixie.' " And Miss Dixie would smile and shoot her hand up.

Besides, I would get behavior reports that the staff might be otherwise reluctant to provide.

"Dixie was on fire today," John would tell me. "En fuego. Sitting on Harvey's lap."

"Arggh," I would groan. "Does Harvey have a wife?"

"Oh yes," he would reply.

Then, later, Miss Dixie's displeasure would be communicated in a cat-like hiss when he moved to take something from her that she was shredding to pieces and messing up his cab with. "She hissed at me," John would say, "like an angry cat."

"Oh yeah, she does that," I said. And then John would talk about the marvelous Metropolitan Opera performance he and his wife had just seen in New York City, or a fabulous recipe he had prepared over the weekend.

*

Then, there was wonderful Mary. "How is Mama Dixie?" Mary asked on the phone. She had taken care of the mother of friends a decade earlier, and she was nothing short of spectacular. Not surprisingly, she was very much in demand, too.

I first met Mary in the late 1980s when she was taking care of Frances Piccolo, the mother of my friends Tito Piccolo and Joann Piccolo Carmody. Mama Piccolo was Italian and a strong personality. She was charming, elegant, and smart. She didn't have Alzheimer's but another neurological disorder that impacted her communication ability. The Piccolos were part of my St. Louis circle when I was growing up. Tito and I went to his Senior Prom together, etc. Neither of us knew that the other was settling in DC. Tito came to Georgetown for graduate school, and we later formed an interior design business called Barti Associates. *Bar. Ti. Get it.*

Anyway, as Mrs. Piccolo, who lived with Tito, got more infirmed, it was essential for him to get some help with his mother, who could be very strong-willed and opinionated. After chasing away and firing a series of agency-vetted people, Mary came to work her magic on Mama Piccolo. All of Tito and Joann's friends learned quickly of Mary's magic. She had a way of gaining confidence and cooperation that was astounding.

When I was first looking for companions, Mary was very busy with her own client base and really was more skilled than I needed at the time. But, there came a time when Mary became available and Miss Dixie's needs were requiring more skill.

Mary walked in the door and start talking and immediately engaging with Miss Dixie. My mother was her total and exclusive attention. Until I saw Mary in action, I didn't realize how unengaged some of our agency help had been. Not the full-time people so much, but those who were substitutes.

Mary would take Mamma Dixie outside to sit on the porch, and Mary would cut the bushes. I'm not kidding. If the rose bushes looked too gangly, Mary would ask for the trimmers and take care of it—all while she was talking with Miss Dixie out on the porch. Mary was that kind of person: a total and complete gem. And, she would call periodically to find out how Mama Dixie was.

Then there was Jay. Jay Dunn from the Alzheimer's group had first saved our bacon by taking apart and putting back together the famous Medicare hospital bed when there was no repair service and Miss Dixie was stuck three feet off the ground.

SERIOUS SNOW AND THE ALZHEIMER'S PATIENT

By December 2009, Jay Dunn needed a place to stay. Jay, another just-in-time caregiving helper, had cared for his mother and father, both of whom had Alzheimer's roughly a decade before I met him at our Alzheimer's support group. He had volunteered to help me if I ever needed it.

He moved into the front part of my house, which, after my dad died, was a space for caregivers, except that I didn't have any caregivers at the time. Our deal was that Jay was to help with yard work and mother's care in exchange for rent. A sweat equity arrangement. So as Northern Virginia began its memorable snow odyssey, fifty-five inches of snow when it typically had fifteen inches, an official snow-shovel person had taken up residence. It was a wonderful thing. The Universe was looking after Mother and me once again.

The first big snowfall started threatening Christmas week. Friends headed for Florida for the holidays quickly changed their reservations and got out of DC while planes were still flying and roads were clear. DC and its surroundings are notoriously wimpy when it comes to snow. Much of the time the anxiety over a little puff of snowy weather will close everything. But, I grew up in serious snow and below-zero weather. In my first year in college in East Lansing, MI, I would walk half a mile to class in three pairs of wool socks, long underwear, jeans, ski pants, two or three wool sweaters, and a ski jacket. Of course, about midway through class, my head was wet from sweating, sitting there in that winter garb. This Christmas-week DC storm was impressive even to me. It was serious snow.

My kitchen in the addition was dark as snow piled up on the skylight. Usually, the wind would blow it off or the sun would melt it quickly. Not this time. The border of bamboo in the backyard was arched to the center with twelve-foot poles loaded with snow. As long as the power stayed on, it was wondrous to watch nature re-sculpt the landscape from the inside.

The media started calling this nor'easter a blizzard. So, it was snow, wind, and no visibility for a while. More than sixteen inches of snow fell at Reagan National Airport. Other parts of Northern Virginia reported twenty-four inches. Everything was shutdown. Transportation, schools, and DAY CARE.

Even though Jay was living in the front of the house, there was privacy. I didn't know he was there until I heard the scrape of the snow shovel. He certainly had his work cut out for him. It was really a tunneling process—a path to the road, then widen the path to clear the driveway. Find the walk in front of the house. Clear it, even though it was unlikely to have travelers immediately after the snow. On and on.

Somewhere along the way, I had started giving Miss Dixie breakfast in bed. Warm oatmeal loaded with cinnamon, raisins, prunes, bananas, and her crushed-up meds. Food started her off on a positive note, and I usually could get her into the shower after that.

So for us, the storm was just like a weekend day. I'd start my day with my exercise bike as I read the news on my laptop and then showered. I no longer walked with a cane or was in pain from my hip. I had had hip replacement surgery. Though I was mobile, I really wasn't up to shoveling snow and taking care of Miss Dixie at the same time. She would sleep a little later, have breakfast. Then I would shower and dress her. I'd put old movies on and we would walk to the family room and kitchen for lunch and conversation. The kitchen was open to the dining table in the family room, so I could work in the kitchen making soup and freezing it while Miss Dixie sat at the table. In the early days, she used to come around the corner into the kitchen to watch me chopping. Not so much now, but we were both grateful for the open space that allowed us to function separately yet be together.

The storm, plus the time off from day care because of the yearend holidays, meant Miss Dixie was home a lot in the last couple weeks of the year. Without car rides as an entertainment option, I was running short on ideas. Miss Dixie was talking a lot. Lots of repetitions. Day care had spoiled me. I was used to Miss Dixie having so much activity at day care that the nonstop repetitive stuff was at a minimum when she was home. Even Miss Dixie was getting bored with our movie selection. It wasn't nearly as entertaining as having volunteer live performers twice a day at day care.

I found myself creating my own "happy place." My mind could wander to my happy place with no serious effort on my part. I would be sitting beside Miss Dixie in our television room, which was also where her hospital bed was. Off in my own la la land, then I would hear a very loud, "Hello? Hello? Is anyone there?" Jarred back to reality and laughing at her understanding of where I was, I answered and wondered if my mind was going more quickly than I expected.

Another time, she announced: "I want you to listen to me before you tell me NO." I listened and said, "No," again.

The snow cleared away enough in January to celebrate Mother's birthday at day care. There was a musician playing that afternoon as we celebrated with a large, delicious carrot cake. Miss Dixie wore a big golden paper crown for her birthday—her ninety-third. I grabbed her winter hat and sat on it so I could take pictures of her without that hat.

The snow kept Jay busy from January to March. It was one storm after another. The temperature never warmed up enough between snowstorms to make much of a dent in the piles of snow. My driveway faced the south, so it usually melted quickly with not much effort on my part. Not this year. We had another nor'easter early in February, followed by another ten inches later in the month. It just kept coming.

Day care closed if the school systems closed. So much snow piled in the road and driveway that there was no safe place for the cab to bring Miss Dixie in, as the schools began re-opening. Desperation was settling in my little brain. I was considering crawling the six miles to day care on my hands and knees with Mother on my back. Seriously. Then came spring.

Religion, Spirituality, and Mysticism

I define myself as a spiritual person who doesn't fit easily into the boxes of organized religion. The God stuff is fine, but I'm a little iffy on the Jesus thing. Sure, I like Christmas and Easter, especially the music. But, I don't consider myself a full-on Christian in the traditional sense. Actually, I blame my relatives in West Virginia for some of my religious reluctance. At the age of four, I was introduced to full-immersion baptism by none other than the Baptist Church. There I was, standing on the banks of a nasty-looking creek peeking through bushes as a grownup woman in a white dress was dunked completely under the water. Dirty, nasty water. Since I did not yet know how to swim, I was ready to run. Plus, I remember lots of loud yelling and shouting. *People, you scared a little kid to death.* My four-year-old eyes could see no reasonable explanation for anything going on there. *Skedaddle*, I said to myself. *Maybe I can find Grandmother.*

The last church I belonged to was the St. Louis (MI) First Methodist Church, probably United Methodist now. Rather than belong, I have since attended Presbyterian, Unitarian, and Episcopal Churches for months and years at a time. The Bryn Mawr (PA) Presbyterian Church had soaring, fabulous music and an aesthetically pleasing sanctuary. The Unitarian Universalist Church in Arlington (VA) had interesting and thoughtful speakers, but I missed the "Christian" words to the familiar music. Just before Miss Dixie came to live with me, I attended St. Columba's Episcopal Church in the District, where the energy, music, and pastoral messages really came together for me. That was my church on 9/11, too.

I discovered meditation in 2000 and added yoga with some study of Buddhism. I'm an Episco-Bu, as my friend Lynne would say. Another friend and colleague might have considered me a little too "New Age" for his Episcopalian tastes, but maybe not. I never thought of myself as a New Age person. In any case, I'm not an atheist. I believe that the Universe has somehow looked after me despite my best efforts to do incredibly stupid things sometimes. But, I have trouble picking one specific box among the religious options. Further, I found that I was turned off by the absolutist tone of many religious types.

Frankly, it amazed me how often the Universe looked in on Miss Dixie and me in our Alzheimer's journey. At several points I felt a need for conversations with God. Beyond that, there were clearly moments when the Universe presented a solution that I had not even considered. What do you call that? I called it grace.

My grace list goes something like this.

Fear not. Alzheimer's should not be feared. A friend at a weekend meditation gathering told me about her experience and her brother's success taking care of her father, an Alzheimer's patient. This piece of information not only lifted my spirits, but also changed everything about the way I thought about caring for my parents.

Keep the music on. My father was in the hospital dying. A new nurse came on for the overnight shift. She read the story of my father's life that I left on the windowsill. It touched her and she promised to keep the music in the boom box going all night. I could take my mother home and put her to bed. My guilt at leaving my father could go on pause as I took care of my other responsibility.

Let it snow. My snow shoveler took up residence in our house the week the snowstorms started. The year of serious, disabling snow became manageable. Further, I didn't have to worry whether the EMTs could get up the driveway if something happened.

Money pains. This was a direct conversation with God, a prayer. My thesis was this: if we do the private pay day care thing, we'll be rolling through cash big time. I will run out of THEIR money. Do I risk my own retirement by tapping into those funds for Miss Dixie's care? I knew my Dad would not want me to risk my future. He was even nervous about my taking on the construction of the addition to my house at my age.

"So God, this is Barbara speaking. What do you think? I don't want to ask for anything specific or too much, but I could use some advice here. I'm feeling a little stuck. Thy will be done."

To my great surprise, my prayer was answered. Miss Dixie's medication was accidentally returned, and with it, her independent mobility returned. She was an anomaly—an Alzheimer's patient who made significant improvement—and was able to return for more than six months to the county-run day care program where fees were based on her modest income. That six months was an unexpected gift. Before it happened, it never, ever occurred to me as a possibility.

Then, the most magnificent of all gifts. The Fed Ex truck pulled up to the house. *What in the world?* I asked myself. *I didn't order anything.* I ripped open the envelope. Inside I found two five-figure checks, one for me and one for my mother. Two checks. Both were signed by Ann L. Bronfman.

Ann had told me years ago, "Let me know if you need 'help.' " Help is that wonderful euphemism that the very rich and highly philanthropic use as the word for money. Janey Hart had said the same thing. Ann and Janey had been friends for more than thirty years. Both were wealthy, but Ann's wealth was greater. Every year for three years the five-figure checks arrived at the beginning of the calendar year. The gifts were tax-free and would be deducted from her estate when Ann died, which ironically happened five months after my mother's death.

What words do you use? How do you thank someone adequately for a gift that transforms your life? Yes, I still worried especially as my own health diminished, but the worry was manageable with Ann's intervention.

Before Ann's gifts began, I had done some consulting work for Ann and her foundation. One year as we were going someplace, she told me she gave away more than a million dollars a year. This was personal money through individual gifts like the ones she made to mother and me. And, it was in addition to the charitable gifts made through her foundation and personally.

So was it magic? Serendipity? Or, the Universe looking out for two folks on an Alzheimer's journey? What was it?

Thy Will Be Done.

And, gratitude forever.

PSYCHOTIC BITCH AND OTHER REGRESSIONS

"And how's Miss Dixie today?" asked my wonderful hair stylist/ friend, Roi Barnard.

"She's a psychotic bitch," I replied.

Caught off-guard, he bent over laughing. "Don't hold back, Barbara," he continued, "tell us what you really think." Roi remembered the stories and even repeated them back to me from time to time. Then, I zoned out to be taken care of. One of my few luxuries for myself.

Miss Dixie's aggression was increasing. It started showing up in reports from day care: aggression in the bathroom, aggression when someone tried to remove her gloves, a plate, or a spoon. It used to be every six weeks or so; now it was every two weeks. I had started noting the days when getting her going in the morning started with aggression. Hitting, kicking, and, this morning, biting. I didn't tell Roi, but my morning with the lovely lady featured her biting me in the breast while I gave her a shower. Of course, it was the breast I had cancer in.

I walked out of the shower. Furious. Mad as hell. I needed five minutes to cool off and change the energy. There didn't seem to be any medication that worked on late-stage aggression without significant risks. We had actually tried the antipsychotic medications at the urging of a day care nurse in the county program. The antipsychotics came with a black box warning that said something like: do not use on older persons; it'll kill them.

Give me some of that stuff, I thought to myself. *Killing an old lady today has some appeal. Deep breaths, Barbara. Deep breaths.*

Eventually, she settled down and we got to day care later than usual, but none the worse for wear. As the disease progressed, it would take twenty minutes and two people to get her out of bed and, later, into the car. Her outbursts were happening more frequently. One Alzheimer's conversation went like this:

Me: "Let's get up, get a shower, and do your hair."

Dixie: "No," said with belligerence. "My feet are down here."

As I tucked Mother into bed that night, she said, "I think I'll stay with you tonight." To which, I replied, "That's good. I'm glad."

*

Part of me was noticing and part of me was denying it. The annoying paradoxes of caregiving were there again.

The nagging reality suggested Miss Dixie was failing. Little things that now I can't even explain, but I knew our time was coming to an end. She knew it, too. In the spring on the way to day care, I would reach over to touch her hand while I was driving and she held my hand. I know it's strange, but I can't tell how much that meant to me. *Such an emotional roller coaster, this family caregiving business.*

In May, at Dad's birthday, probably, I was reminded of his death and how emotionally unprepared I had been. Grant did a moving eulogy, but I felt badly that I had not gotten myself together enough to write one, too. I really wanted to do a eulogy for my mother. So, in May I started writing. A little bit here and there, since I knew it would be so difficult to consider after she was gone.

In late May, I was also surprised by the death of Miss Dixie's youngest brother, Russell. He had diabetes and Alzheimer's. Diabetes seems to mean a greater likelihood of getting Alzheimer's, according to research data, but the connection is still vague.[22] The experience of the Garrett family pointed to inconsistency in the connection, also. Uncle Loman, who was still alive then, had had diabetes for years and no Alzheimer's. And Miss Dixie had no diabetes, but had Alzheimer's.

22. Mayo Clinic Staff, "Diabetes and Alzheimer's Linked," Mayo Clinic, April 3, 2013, accessed August 13, 2015, http://www.mayoclinic.org/diseases-conditions/alzheimers-disease/in-depth/diabetes-and-alzheimers/art-20046987.

One Colossal Failure and Other Challenges

It was the stuff that wasn't Alzheimer's specifically that presented the greater challenges. The surprises included the following: urinary tract infections (UTIs); skin ulcers on her toes and heels, her calf and ankle, and the worst from the rubbing of her adult diaper between her legs; and her teeth.

Her teeth were my colossal failure.

In the early stages, I thought Miss Dixie's teeth, which were good, would not be on my list of problems. I remembered spending time with the wife of an Alzheimer's caregiving support group member who had no teeth. It made me sad to see her. She looked like an Alzheimer's patient, and I didn't want my mother to have the look. *I would hate for my mother to lose her teeth,* I said to myself. By the time we reached the advanced stages, I viewed the issue entirely differently.

Right after she was diagnosed with Alzheimer's, I spent $3,000 getting her teeth fixed after a couple of years of neglected dental care and lost dental bridges. I resolved not to make that kind of investment again, but I never envisioned the dental care problems that we experienced in later stages.

In fact in 2004 and 2005, I was delighted that I was able to teach her to use an electric toothbrush with assistance. She not only used it willingly, but also seemed to enjoy it.

The first dentist I took Mother to was a mistake. Since he was also my dentist, I took her with me to my appointment in the early stages. While I was in the chair, Mother didn't like the energy in the office. She was right about that. So, Miss Dixie got up, put her hat and coat on, and left. Yes, the office staff knew she had Alzheimer's, but... Not helpful. That particular day the office was staffed by the dentist's wife, too.

So, I returned to the waiting room to find her gone. I went into panic mode and tore out of the office. She was walking around the parking lot looking at the trees. Once I got over the terror of her being missing, I had to laugh. She was absolutely right. The energy in that place said: get out of here.

I thought I was taking care of Mother's teeth as best I could. Brushing twice a day. Dental visits three times a year. In the late stages, those mouth muscles locked and it took forever to coax a toothbrush through her mouth. I tried every technique, every trick, but nothing worked. I attended classes dealing with teeth and dental care. My mother's beautiful, well-cared-for teeth disappeared in the depths of Alzheimer's, and I failed to communicate effectively with dental care providers. I thought I had made it clear. I wanted cavities taken care of, but no, I was not going for crowns and high-dollar repairs. Our new dentist, recommended by the Alzheimer's Association, seemed to think I was content to let her teeth fall out. That was not my intention. In the months before Mother's death I was pursuing a new dental strategy. I had asked a friend, Barry Cooper, who had been a caregiver and who knew far more than I did about dental issues, to help me think through what needed to be done. I took her for a second opinion to a dentist who had been a nurse practitioner. I was looking at hospitalizing her and putting her under an anesthetic for dental work. I was sure there was infection lurking somewhere. And, infection anywhere was a serious matter in the frail elderly.

At that point, I thought about prophylactic extraction of teeth early in the disease as a "best practices" course of action. Yes, I would have hated the look. Would she have lived longer? Who knows? There are no best practices for Alzheimer's. And, I should add here that no one else seems to think of extraction as a recommended approach. Those tightened muscles and the resistance from my advanced stage Alzheimer's patient still torture me in hindsight. I don't see options and other possibilities for dental care. Yet, I'm convinced it is extremely important.

*

One of the myths that I bought into was that skin ulcers would not occur if the patient was not bedridden or in a wheelchair. Unfortunately, with experience as my teacher, I learned that skin ulcers could occur, be nasty, and be hard to treat, even if the patient was fairly mobile and not bedridden.

As a non-medical and non-scientific person, I gathered that skin ulcers and bedsores, also called pressure sores, were similar. A web search turned up more quality information on bedsores than skin ulcers. Using the Mayo Clinic symptom stages,[23] Miss Dixie's feet were stage I; her calf and thigh sores were stage II. At the time, it seemed to me that the thigh sore, in particular, was more serious than a stage II lesion, but perhaps it was just my anxiety about the location and difficulty keeping it clean.

An inexpensive, five-dollar, topical medication was used on her toes and heels, at first with regular drug store bandages, and then as it improved, medication without bandages. With the calf lesion we graduated to non-stick bandages, the topical medication, and an antibiotic.

With the thigh lesion, we became patients of the wound care center, which turned out to be a wonderful resource. What a wonderful discovery that place was. In addition to cultures on the spot, they had fabulous bandages that covered the spot and stayed on for days. Even Miss Dixie couldn't take it off. After a couple of weeks, we returned to the center to have the bandage changed and new topical medication applied. Then, we got to the hard part. I was supposed to change the bandage and apply the medication, which cost more than $140 for a very small supply. I simply didn't have enough hands to keep Miss Dixie from hitting and pushing me away to pull this off on my own. So, the fix for this problem was a visiting nurse. I probably lost a couple of months off my own lifespan with this episode and the anxiety it produced.

*

Urinary tract infections (UTIs) have been present at some point in the disease continuum with every Alzheimer's patient I've heard of and many older, non-Alzheimer's individuals. They can be particularly nasty. To the uninitiated in the care of older folks as I was, an infection means a fever. Not true with a urinary tract infection in the elderly. The patient can be very, very ill without a fever. Symptoms can mimic Alzheimer's with greater disorientation, confusion, etc., and as we learned repeatedly, the first antibiotic prescribed may not work. A new one was often prescribed after the culture was analyzed. A urinary tract infection was hard work

---

23. Mayo Clinic Staff, "Bedsores (pressure sores): Symptoms," Mayo Clinic, December 13, 2014, http://www.mayoclinic.org/diseases-conditions/bedsores/basics/symptoms/con-20030848.

for me. Miss Dixie could not self-report, and she couldn't pee in a cup. So, I had to get the patient to a place where a catheter could be inserted. Often, she couldn't walk by the time the infection became obvious. And on and on.

These issues were the most significant ongoing challenges of our journey. In between, there were cataract surgeries and minor skin cancer surgeries. Bandages that were supposed to stay on were ripped off immediately. Etcetera, etcetera. Still, we were lucky. Other folks had more serious heart, cancer, or arthritis issues.

Very often, pneumonia starts the beginning of the final downward slide. That was the case with Miss Dixie, but I was still so obsessed with keeping her alive that it didn't register with me. The lesson from all of this? Alzheimer's makes the routine health stuff at least twice as hard, sometimes more. Have courage and carry on! And, when it's over, don't beat yourself up for not "getting it" sooner. Though "it" is different with all of us, denial helps us put one foot in front of the other. And that may be useful to the caregiver's mental wellbeing!

Friday Night in the ER

Off in the distance, I heard sirens. *I hope those aren't our sirens.* But, of course, they were. In a matter of minutes, the rescue unit and the fire truck from Falls Church pulled up in front of the neighbor's house and backed up to our house. A group of hardy young men, maybe six, bounded from the trucks and up the driveway that late August evening.

"Are you the patient?" the first one asked. "Oh, no, inside," I said.

Miss Dixie was slumped over on a bedside toilet. Thoughts of privacy and modesty were replaced as my desperation as a caregiver increased and the physical difficulty of care giving grew. It would never, ever have occurred to me that I would have allowed my mother to be seen on the toilet by men and the world several years ago, but here I was. Keeping my mother alive with some quality of life was my priority and one of the blessings of Alzheimer's was that SHE would not remember a thing, including her humiliation if she had been unencumbered by Alzheimer's.

The EMTs struggled to arouse her. Unresponsive. "Was she always like this?" they asked me.

"No, she has had a slight fever (100.2) for two days now. The only other symptom that I can find is a nasty cough, so it sounds like some kind of bronchial thing to me, and, of course, I'm worried about pneumonia."

"Was she having a bowel movement on the toilet?"

"I don't know," I said. Turned out she was, and sometimes she blacked out when she had a bowel movement. I didn't discover all of this until the ambulance left the house. I headed to my computer, looking for the list of medications I made for fast access in ER situations. Of course, it wasn't fast. I couldn't find it. Anxiety, stress, whatever made the search difficult.

I found a file, but not "the" file. Good enough. Copied her Medicare and gap insurance cards. They were off. I changed my clothes, turned the fire off from under the chili pot, picked up my current book for a long evening of waiting and reading, and headed to the ER. I had learned that it took them awhile to get settled into a cubicle in the ER, so I didn't break my neck trying to get there. But I also didn't dawdle.

I've never met a first responder who wasn't terrific. They were well-trained and related well to both the patient and the caregiver, which wasn't always the case with other medical personnel. There was often a level of indifference from medical office staff. I was sure it wasn't intended, but it was there.

When I arrived at the ER I was able to walk right in to Cubicle Seven. The EMT was there finishing his computer report. Since I had cleaned Mother's toilet before I left, I mentioned that she sometimes passed out on the toilet, but returned to be herself in about twenty minutes.

"Oh yes," he said, "the (something) nerve." Most other health care providers usually looked at me as if I had three heads when I said she blacked out. Then, they proceeded to explain to me that blacking out probably wasn't good for the patient. *No kidding. It wasn't easy on the caregiver either.* But, sometimes it happened.

I took comfort from one report from my support group of an Alzheimer's patient who fainted a couple of times a year. The medical folks never could identify a cause, so why try to explain it to a doctor or a nurse—just deal with it when it happens. That way you can ignore the anxiety in the provider's voice. Their anxiety messed with my karma. But, these EMT guys got it. They must see it frequently with frail older people.

"Boy, she's really strong," the EMT continued. "Ripped the IV connection right out."

"Yeh," I said. "And she kicks. Hits and *bites* by way of a warning."

So, Mother's tests in the ER required triple teaming. Since she no longer could be counted on to respond to verbal commands, "relax" meant nothing to her. I mentioned that to a tech and he retorted, "I have to say something to her." *Okay, knock yourself out. Just don't expect her to do what you want.* Eventually, he got the drift and went with the triple team plan.

"She spits, too," a member of the catheter team reported as she exited Mother's cubicle. I was smart enough to leave the room for that one.

Wailing babies. One drunk or addict who had a full security detail provided by the hospital was trying to break the sound barrier. After he was situated in a cubicle, I only heard him scream for an apple. I didn't wait around to see if he got one. Chest X-ray, blood work, and finally about five hours later, Miss Dixie and I headed to a room. Actually, the population of the ER seemed sparse compared to previous visits. Loud, but sparse.

The new hospital wing very thoughtfully allowed family members a sofa bed to stay over. I didn't stay over this time, because my sanity required that I restore some order to my surroundings just in case Mother didn't come home soon.

Maybe it sounds crazy, but bringing a little order seemed to help me cope. It felt like I was doing something constructive and that I was in control, which was so untrue. By the way, control freaks usually do not do well as hands-on caregivers. Most of the time I was a roll-with-it type. So, I started emptying my huge chili pot. Refrigerator. Freezer. The recipe made at least twenty servings. Finished the laundry. Started the dishwasher. Cleaned the kitchen counters and cooktop. Let people know what was going on by email. Before polyurethane, I used to wax floors when my anxiety level was off the charts. Now, I make large quantities of healthy, largely vegetarian soup. When everything else was reeling, I took some comfort in knowing we would have healthy stuff available to eat. That was my coping drill.

*

Always, too, I would think about my mother. Caregivers are protectors. It starts with keeping the person safe from harm. Then, it kind of morphed into keeping the person safe from hurt feelings, especially in the early days. In early Alzheimer's, it can't be assumed that the patient won't get it. More things register. The patient remembers more. Caregivers start assuming responsibility for protecting feelings. Hurt feelings from insensitive, snarky remarks. Incompetence. Indifference. The list grows, all by itself. Responsibility for the cocoon of care and protection. A bonding against the brutality of the disease.

In the early years, Dixie had shared a lot of information. Still, I believed there were secrets from her childhood hidden away. She could be very prudish. She said that she knew nothing about sex until she married. How could that be, growing up on a farm? It just didn't fit. My dad thought she hid things because as a child her male cousins from down the road would roar through the house and take her belongings. He characterized the cousins as ornery to delinquent. One of their favorite things was to throw black snakes into the car as he was driving to pick Mother up for a date. Was there more that her rowdy tormentors did? I didn't find out before Alzheimer's. Now I would never know. Secrets and reasons would forever remain a mystery.

As her release from the hospital rolled around, I failed to plan well. I failed miserably. I thought I could handle getting her out of the car by myself. Wrong. Really dumb on my part. She had transferred into the car okay. But, getting out was something else. I pulled into the driveway. Still not thinking about what could happen. I looked to see if Jay was around. He wasn't. No reason for him to be. I put this terrific special gait belt around her. It had handles and everything. Midway through the transfer from the car to the wheelchair I knew I was in big trouble. She was dead weight. And, I still wasn't able to get leverage to move her.

She was halfway out of the car and I panicked. This was not going to work. I had my purse on top of the car. I grabbed my cell phone and called Tito. Thank heavens he was home.

"I've made a huge mistake and I need help as fast as you can get here," I said. Within minutes he was there.

"Okay, we need to plan this," he said. "Which way are we going and who's doing what?"

Eventually we got her into the house and into bed. *I swear that hour and a half aged me six months.*

Voodoo Hand Dance

The August hospitalization set Miss Dixie back. A nursing assistant came to help at home before she could return to day care. It took two of us to get her moving every day. She was still taking antibiotics for pneumonia. Her walking was sketchy; sometimes she could walk, sometimes she couldn't. So, our physical therapist Joni also came to help. There was no way I could handle her without some level of mobility. In denial again, I was refusing to face the future of her care. One foot in front of the other. The future was too complicated. A friend brought his caregiving mechanical lift. The nursing assistant and I tried it. Miss Dixie pushed us away. She couldn't understand what needed to happen. No cooperation. Transfers between the bed and wheelchair were horrific. So much of the time she was not only dead weight, but also fighting every movement.

Subconsciously, the terror was setting in. I would not be able to care for her at home much longer. I would fail in my promise to my father and mother. I would fail. *No, no. Let's keep trying. There must be a way.*

She had been out of day care about a month, long enough that she required a new assessment to return. I was anxious that she might not do well, but she passed. In October, she could return.

Still, I was restless and unsettled about the future.

*

The phone rang. I was expecting Miss Dixie to arrive by taxi from day care. Caller ID said it was John D, our Red Top cab driver.

"I'm out in front. Could you bring the wheelchair out?" John asked. Sometimes Mother was tired from walking these days, and the portable wheelchair was our solution. I usually used it at night to take her down the hall to dinner. I rolled out the back door and rounded the corner to the driveway. *Whoa. What's this?*

John and Miss Dixie were both seated on the blacktop of the road braced up against the cab. Miss Dixie was distressed, but I couldn't tell whether it was pain or fear. It took two of us lifting to get her into to the wheelchair amid excruciating cries of anguish from Miss Dixie. Again, was it fear or pain?

As we rolled her in the house, John told me what had happened. He was helping her out of the cab when Miss Dixie became dead weight. I knew that feeling of dead weight. I had felt it when I tried to get her out of the car in August. It seemed to happen in mid-transfer. Terrified, I had called Tito to come help me. There was no gait belt in the world that would have helped that solo transfer.

Now, I'm not sure why, but I decided to wait a little while to see if she settled down after the cab incident. We had been through this scene so many times. Call the ambulance, go to the ER, wait, get some X-rays, and wait some more. It was just six weeks since her last trip to the ER. Did we really need to go this time?

I waited a while just to see if she settled down. She didn't. Maybe it was something serious. I called for transport help. This time there were no sirens. *Did they know the house? Maybe. Apparently.* One of the EMTs remarked as he arrived that he had been at the house before.

The emergency room was much quieter this trip. Once she was stretched out in bed, she dozed off to sleep. As she prepared to go for X-rays, both the ER doc and I noted that an X-ray was probably an exercise in excessive caution. Her anguish was gone; she seemed peaceful. She was taken to X-ray by one person; this time I didn't have to go with her. I settled into to Room Five and its cream-colored privacy curtain to read my book while I waited. I noted soft blue, green, and gray geometric patterns. Were they fabrics, wall coverings, or flooring? I don't know. I do know they provided a pleasant, soothing feeling that was strong enough for me to notice and remember.

An hour later, the X-ray report was in. Not a false alarm. Fractured femur. Up we went to the seventh floor. I could see the full moon and the treetops below. It was a beautiful, crisp fall evening, a contrast of tranquility to my growing anxiety about my mother. Surgery might come the next day. Mother rested comfortably. I decided to go home. I knew I would be staying over during and after surgery. I would need to have my wits about me. I needed rest.

Her fall, I kept thinking about her fall. Replaying it in my head. She was doing so well. Back in day care. I had been making plans for her to stay in day care and was applying for a discount based on income to slow down the churning through cash. As I look back on that period of time, I believe I was experiencing a kind of progression denial. Part of me understood that she was getting worse, but part of me was holding on to the status quo for dear life. Even though her day care program would accept late-stage patients, did day care still really make sense? For her, maybe. For me? Probably not. It was killing me to get her there. In retrospect, I think I was in denial. But that never occurred to me as I was going through it. For two months now, it took two people to get her up in the morning. The risk of falling was terrifying, but I still kept pushing to keep her moving and to keep her in day care. Instead, was it time for me to think about her being a largely bedridden patient? Somehow I couldn't wrap my head around that idea.

Then, once we got her up and showered and dressed, the next contest was getting her in and out of the car. She had taken to refusing to get out of the car to go in to day care. It could easily take twenty minutes to try to coax her into cooperation. Sometimes I had to ask for help from the day care staff. Why was I going through this? I never stopped to ask myself that question. It was what I had always done so I would still do it. *Think, Barbara, think.* No time for thinking. I needed her to be in day care so I could go to the dentist and the doctor. This was what I saw in hindsight, not as it was happening.

Her surgery on the femur was delayed as they pumped her full of antibiotics. A urinary tract infection. I worried about an infection also coming from her teeth, which had become a serious problem in the last six months. Getting her teeth fixed moved to the back burner with her new injury. Now in the hospital she slept all the time, but I stayed over when I thought surgery might be early in the morning. It wasn't. Still, the hospital had a sofa for family sleepovers. How different from the misery of stiff chairs when my dad was hospitalized.

In the early morning hours, a technician came in to take vital signs. It was quite something to watch. English was a second language for the tech; she would tell the patient what she was doing. That meant nothing to Miss Dixie, of course. At first, I tried to explain, "Alzheimer's. She doesn't understand." The tech didn't get it or ignored me, I'm not sure which. Then, I watched in full amusement as my mother scared her off and ran her out of the room.

Miss Dixie turned into a Caribbean witch doctor. Both hands flew through the air at the same time as though she was dispensing voodoo, fingers and wrists shaking and flying. I chuckled. She could still take care of herself on some level. If Miss Dixie didn't want to do it, it wasn't going to happen. The tech left without the odious vital signs.

*

The blood pressure cuff had always been her most hated piece of medical equipment. She yelled, wiggled, and begged for it to stop. Occasionally she would try something more violent, but she also knew when to back off. Once, when she was in the hospital, her doctor took her blood pressure. I happened to not be in the room. Miss Dixie complained. When it was over, she said resolutely but quietly to the doctor, "I want you to leave." Somehow, Miss Dixie knew this was someone not to be hit or kicked. This person had a certain kind of presence. A persona and white jacket. So Miss Dixie behaved. Afterward, her doctor told me about it with a smile and a chuckle.

Visits to the podiatrist were another matter. The podiatrist was terrific. His office was in an old Arlington house. There wasn't much square footage on the lot. The county wouldn't let him put in a ramp for disabled patients, so he made house calls for his wheelchair patients. He came to see us at the house on Sundays, too. Our first home visit was after a hospitalization in 2007 when Miss Dixie was not yet able to walk. Later, she was able to walk and she returned to the office.

Both of her feet were disasters. She had a hammertoe on one foot and skin ulcers on various toes and heels. Bandages and medication were part of our daily maintenance program. I absolutely could not trim her toenails. (Her fingernails were equally a nightmare that I wrestled with on my own.) Her feet needed special care. The podiatrist visits were wild adventures. I would get Miss Dixie into the chair, which she didn't like particularly. There were minor protests like, "Let's go." But we didn't.

I don't think there was ever a word exchanged between the doctor and me, but I held her arms and her legs while he worked. She screamed and screamed. Both the podiatrist and I pretended not to notice. The office was small enough that his waiting room patients could certainly hear. Years ago, my conduct and the fact that people could hear would have bothered me. But not now. You just did what you had to do. When the doctor was finished, Miss Dixie had no pent-up anger. She was happy again as I put her socks and shoes on. And, off we went to day care or home for lunch.

At other appointments, doctors were always late, sometimes very late. There were risks making old people wait. In the beginning, I shouldered the anxiety of the risks. After a while I started to see the result as a justification for the wait. Adult diapers were good, but not perfect. Sometimes the fit was off or they got overloaded. When I noticed a spot of dampness on an office chair after an hour's wait, I came to not care. In fact, a secret smile. *Happens when you're late.*

So, her voodoo hand dance in the hospital was just another one of her theatrical numbers. Her repertoire of self-care.

As daylight came to the hospital, nursing shifts changed and the sounds of bustling activity took over. I slipped out to go home for a shower. When I returned, Miss Dixie's doctor was finishing up and a social worker asked to see me. Surgery was to be delayed because of the infection, but after surgery the social worker was recommending hospice care at home. Don't ask me why, but I wasn't quite prepared for this particular hospice care discussion. Hospice meant the end. I had trouble grasping it.

MY MOTHER'S ADVICE

In my years of care for my mother, the pressure of one foot in front of the other had meant I had forgotten or misplaced the good advice she had given me before Alzheimer's. I was independent—to a fault, some would say. She would tell me, "Don't settle for any marriage." Was my mother saying she had settled? At one time, her message might have been that she had settled. But, as they grew older as a couple, their love became visibly stronger. She had dreams, only a few of which came true. Now, I could say the same thing of myself. Only a few of my dreams had come true. My father wanted a home and was more contented with a simple life than she was. I probably came close to living the life she dreamed of. Yet, as I aged, I missed what she had. *Funny how that works.* She knew my father took care of her, and she knew she would be in trouble without him. I was alone and an only.

I knew she wanted grandchildren, but to her credit she never, ever said that to me. She taught me to love thunderstorms when I was a child. We huddled on the bed and she told me how wonderful thunder was, masking her terror. She had lots of trouble with her feelings of an empty nest when I went away to college, but I only knew it from former colleagues, who would see her working late in the windows of the dry cleaners. They told me. She didn't tell me.

My mother made me take typing in high school. "You just never know," she had said. My hand-eye coordination was pitiful. On timed tests, I would occasionally break fifty words per minute. Most of the time, I was the rock bottom of the class. I aced the written tests if I didn't have to type. The teacher had me perform typing skits for extra credit when it was her turn to put together an all-school assembly. That's the only way I got through the class.

Dixie was of her generation, but also ahead of her time in her belief that women should be equal. When I was a kid she told me: "Be a doctor, not a nurse. Nurses have to carry bedpans." That memory made me laugh out loud. How many times I would have loved the convenience of a bedpan. I didn't have the chops to be a doctor; a good one, anyway. Yet, I had spent the last ten years of my life doing what she told me not to do. Being a nurse and an advocate for her wellbeing. The crazy thing was I was pretty good at it. Even crazier, I wanted to do it. I believed it was every bit as important as anything else I had done. Here and there some of her messages got screwed up a little bit, but mostly they were solid. So, my reaction to hospice now was odd.

Three years earlier I had done an intake interview with a different hospice provider. That was then, but for some reason I didn't think Miss Dixie was ready for it now. Did hospice mean giving in? Giving in, that the end was near? Despite the risks associated with Miss Dixie's surgery, I was sure she would pull through. Once again, the truth was: My mother was ready for hospice, but I was not.

REMEMBERING MY MODEL CAREGIVER

I went looking for my journal from nearly thirty years earlier, 1981. Lucille was my Alzheimer's caregiving model. I needed to remember her story again as I lived my own.

*

My mother's sister, Lucille, was determined to take care of Grandmother and Granddad, and she did. Grandmother died from Alzheimer's. Lucille's wish to be spared, to allow her to care for her parents, was granted. Despite her treatment for stage IV cancer, Lucille met each hurdle, each challenge, and calmed it—for a time, at least.

Two years passed. It was the middle of April 1981, and I hadn't talked to my mother in at least ten days. It was busy at the office.

Troubling news. Lucille was in the hospital in West Virginia. Her condition had been critical, and it remained not so good. Blood clots on the lungs. A new fluid medicine, it was speculated, might have caused an adverse drug reaction. A blood cell deviation and low hemoglobin was mentioned. Leukemia was one of the potential risks to radiation, Lucille's radiation at least. I said otherwise. Denial. I knew at this conversation that it was leukemia.

Two days later my mother called with a report.

"It's leukemia, isn't it," I said.

"Yes," she said. "The acute kind. But Hopkins has a treatment program." Lucille would be flown by air ambulance to Johns Hopkins— the source of two previously successful rounds with cancer.

May 2, 1981. Midnight. Good news. Lucille arrived at Hopkins Hospital in Baltimore and tests were under way. The first scan was negative. No evidence of Lucille's previous cervical cancer. My mother in Michigan and I in Virginia were euphoric. This week's fight, day by day, was successful. When I had visited Lucille in April I was stunned by how frail she looked. Her brother Herbert, the go-to-person for everything important, died two years ago so the family support model has changed. It seemed I was next in line. Time for me to step up.

I fell asleep again at 6 a.m. Sleep was fitful; I was tired. Nasty-looking clothes. Baggy pants and running shoes. Only essential errands. Got to the bank before it closed. Picked up prescriptions. Put gas in the car. My office was driving me nuts, I told myself. That's why I was so tired. I needed to settle in and get a handle on that stuff in my briefcase. *I think I'll call Lucille and tell her I'm tired. See if she's...*

"When are you coming up?"

"I was kind of thinking of not coming."

"A doctor's coming in to talk with me and I want you here."

"When?"

"Call the nurses' station and ask them, will you? Get on it, huh!"

The doctor's conference was set to happen between 2 and 4 p.m., the nurse reported. I bolted for the car. Who cared what I looked like.

At Hopkins, Room 267, Oncology Two South, I tapped and went in.

"You're up. Terrific," I said. Roll of the eyes from Lucille.

The nurse was helping with Lucille's food tray and reported, "You just missed the excitement. The blood bag broke. Blood all over. Four of us came running."

"Missed the ceiling," I said after a quick glance up.

"Liked to scared me to death," Lucille said. Another roll of the eyes. "When did you talk to your mother last?"

"Midnight," I said.

"She's gonna own the phone company," said Lucille. *Don't I wish.*

After the nurse left, she began, "I talked with a doctor this morning and she was blunt." Her voice was low. I strained to hear. The boisterous, unrestrained vitality of the six-foot Lucille was no longer.

"She said my chances weren't good." I listened intently. Quietly. I knew why I was there. All afternoon we talked and listened to each other, mostly in a shorthand that did not require finished thoughts or sentences. The human connection was extraordinary. I had never experienced anything as deeply connected yet mystical. I would start a sentence; Lucille would finish it and vice versa.

There was a decision to be made. Lucille would make it and she was working it through. Conscious and unconscious measuring.

*

Johns Hopkins, the next day.

Lucille was in bed. A doctor, a resident, I surmised, was working on her. Both forearms were swollen. I saw only an IV bottle. No blood platelets today.

"They were having trouble with veins yesterday," I said, but I was really asking.

"Phlebitis," the doctor responded. Her forearms were to rest, and the IV was attached to her upper chest.

The doctor's conference, delayed one day, began.

Cindy, Lucille's nurse for the day, attended the conference, too. The reason, the doctor explained, was the nurses didn't know why anyone would want to go through this particular treatment. And, they wanted to make sure all parties understood the potential dire effects. The nurses' perspective registered only momentarily with me. Yet, I remembered the rooms of gaunt, bald human beings I had seen on the hospital corridor. I was reminded of images of men and women from World War II. Walking cadavers.

Three drugs were to be used in treatment, the doctor said. I was writing, but I made a mental note to find out what the names of the drugs were later. We discussed what they did. What the side effects were. And, what the periods of isolation would be because of the susceptibility to infection.

There would be time to make the decision, the doctor said. We could call Candace and Kate to talk and think it over. There was no pressure.

Often, the doctor said, the family would say treatment was the decision when the patient didn't want it. That was another reason the nurses wanted to be in the room as the decision was being considered. Too, some patients don't want family around during treatment.

I nodded. "Lucille and I talked yesterday about who in the family should come," I said. "And, I think what we need to know is enough about the treatment so we know who and when."

"But maybe we should ask whether she wants family here." The doctor's words made me wonder if Lucille might have changed her mind.

I asked. The doctor joined in the request.

"Oh my goodness, yes. I want family here," Lucille responded. "No, I don't want to go through it alone."

Well, that took care of that. Cindy had to leave. She said she'd be around for any questions all afternoon. I nodded, knowing we'd have them.

We talked more. Then it happened.

Out of the blue: "No." The answer was no. The doctor had posed the question.

My stomach turned. I was startled. Dazed. Shocked.

My insides screamed. *No. Lucille, no. Fight.*

"No, that isn't life," or something similar is what Lucille had said. The answer was clearly no.

Think about it, the doctor said. And, the family can call me at home. Later Kate would remember the doctor's description: "We will take her to death's door. If she survives, we'll bring her back."

There would be no changing Lucille's decision. It was made.

*

Oh no, now I have to tell the others. I started to make the calls, the horrible calls.

Later. Lucille was dozing. After Kate, Candace, and my mother, Dixie—I quit calling. Others in the family would be calling her today. I would tell them as they called in. I was feeling crazy, sick to my stomach.

Wait a minute. Aunt Maudie. I absolutely had to call her. I had to call her before she came to the hospital. She needed to know before she walked in.

"Did you talk with your mother?" Lucille was awake but I was not ready for her.

"Yes," I said, turning away. I didn't want her to see my tears.

"How'd she take it?"

My mother had demanded to talk with Lucille. I said no. She had sobbed with a wail that was primal in its loss. But I needed to keep her away from Lucille at that moment.

"Bad," I said. My voice sounded funny, and I turned so she couldn't see my face. "Not good." I tried to get my voice straightened out. Still turned away. She shouldn't see me cry. I must not do that to her.

"Did she cry?" Lucille asked.

"Yes," I said. If I didn't say something glib about my mother's crying, Lucille would read me. She read me and stopped talking. Dozing or pretending, I didn't know.

I escaped downstairs. To pull myself together. And make two more calls.

Back in the room, I found Cindy hunkered near the bed holding Lucille's hand. Cindy was saying all of the right things, the things I didn't have the ability to say to Lucille because I didn't want her to see me cry.

"Cindy says I'm courageous," Lucille said with a tone of joy that was almost childlike in its innocence and need. It was so true, so much of what I should be saying. I felt so inadequate.

"Yes, you are," I responded.

Invincible Lucille. In that brief exchange with Cindy, it seemed that she feared she was giving up. It was beyond my capacity to provide the reassurance she needed to hear. I regretted my shortcomings, but I also realized that I had been invited to share in life's most significant decision, to help someone decide to live or die. Advance work for Lucille's journey to the other side, the most important decision we ever make. To live? Or, to die?

"Did you get your mother settled down?" she asked. *How did she know?* Later I would wonder if Lucille hadn't chosen me just to "handle" my mother.

"Did you talk with Maudie?" *How did she know?* The precise two calls that I made. *How DID she know?*

How long did Lucille have to live? "Let's say July 4th, a few weeks," the doctor had said. She added, "There were still miracles." I said that over and over. There were moments when I believed it. Invincible Lucille.

At home, again I looked up Elizabeth Kubler-Ross' five stages of dying: denial, anger, bargaining, depression, and acceptance.

*

A day later. "Lucille, I have no reason to believe it has, but has your decision changed?" My question was by phone. I had to ask.

"No," came the answer softer, lacking the firmness and clarity of the previous day. *Depression*, I said to myself.

I wanted to say again how courageous I thought her decision was. I knew it; I felt it; I wanted to say it. But I would cry. Again, I worried about what she should hear from me, and my inadequacy at providing it. I also remembered the visual assault of the living cadavers. Her decision must not be undermined.

The cheerful tone of my voice worried me. Yet, cheer was the mask I needed to wear. In truth I welcomed that I couldn't be at the hospital today. Later, guilt about that feeling would be something to live with. In her presence, I could not face the thought of losing her. I was durable and had seen some sorrow and suffering. Yet, I couldn't face that the end was near in her presence. I had never helped someone die. I was thirty-eight years old; it was counter intuitive to my experience base.

*

The vigil began. Days later, the first Alzheimer's family caregiver that I ever knew was gone. Once again, I was reminded of this life-changing experience as an advance person for the end-of-life. It gave me comfort thirty years later. I could do this again.

THE DREADED DECISION

Back at Virginia Hospital Center, several hours later, I had talked my way to a comfort level on hospice. The social worker was convincing. Of the list of hospice providers in the area, one offered twenty-four hour care as end-of-life care. I chose that provider based on the recommendation of the social worker, who had worked with them in Florida for her own family. As the patient needed more care coming closer to death, this provider would be present around the clock. Medicare allowed such assistance, but few hospice groups were set up for twenty-four hour staffing levels.

"It sounded very good," I said, "despite the fact that my mother probably will pull out of it and not need the care." *Yeah sure, Barbara.* If that were the case, I was assured that hospice care could be terminated.

One of the odd things I realize now is that I somehow got it into my head that I expected my mother to live to be ninety-five. Her ninety-fourth birthday was three months away, so it wasn't completely unreasonable. I really wanted her to have a ninety-fifth birthday party. Yes, I took it one day at a time, and that was what got me through. But I was also tricking myself with these little intermediate goals. Always looking for reasons to celebrate for Miss Dixie and, let's be honest, for me. I knew that I would lose her, but the intermediate stuff pushed the big loss out further. *Away for a while at least.* That's how I see it now, but didn't at the time. That helped give context to my initial resistance to hospice care when she left the hospital.

She would survive this surgery despite its risk. I was sure. She would celebrate her ninety-fifth birthday. Suppose she survived the surgery and the broken femur healed. What then? I pushed that thought out of my mind. I asked the surgeon to draw me a picture of the break. He did and it looked awful, much tougher than my hip replacement. But she would make it. I was sure. What in blazes was I going to do in eight weeks? How was I going to care for her as a bedridden patient? The questions would pass through my consciousness and I would push them aside. One day at a time I would repeat to myself. *Can't think about that right now.*

*

At last: surgery day. The time kept changing throughout the day. The hospital chaplain stopped by the room as Miss Dixie slept and I waited. We had a delightful conversation about faith, servant leadership, and its surprisingly beneficial gifts. He said something like, "Well, you've been doing that for several years now, haven't you."

I thanked him and said, "Yes." How many years had it taken for me to be able to acknowledge something like that. The mantra I heard in my mother's voice for years was, "don't brag." A generational thing? I've always thought so. My generation was so beaten down that the future generations swung too far to the other side, producing the entitlement folks that no one can stand.

The chaplain's affirmation was greatly appreciated, and after the fact I quietly celebrated my progress into healthy personhood. I could accept and agree with his compliment.

Finally, the transport team arrived to take Miss Dixie to surgery. I followed since she could not answer questions about who she was. A dour, grave-looking anesthesiologist arrived to tell me what a high risk the patient was. *Seriously, I pretty much had the drift on that.* The Scottish Warrior Princess was tempted, but behaved. He seemed to shift out of the picture. I wasn't sure why. Risk averse? Easy to hand off to someone else? Maybe.

The nurse in the pre-operative area arrived. She was an attractive woman with a great cut and style to her salt-and-pepper hair. The prep area was for orthopedic surgery. The nurse, perhaps of Middle Eastern extraction, had simple, very good quality jewelry; especially her earrings, understated and classy, but not the kind that one usually sees on working hospital staff. Definitely not costume jewelry. Her queries suggested that she was obsessive-compulsive about her checklist but had some problems remembering whether she had asked the questions before. Still, her most noticeable feature was her back. She was stooped to an eighty-degree, almost ninety degree angle. Here we were, waiting for orthopedic surgery with a medical professional who seemed to exemplify an orthopedic failure. *Not exactly a confidence builder*, mumbled the Scottish Warrior Princess.

Then in came a nurse in charge of paperwork. English was clearly her second language, but she had a good command of it nonetheless. "Surgery could not continue," she announced, "because the hospital did not have a copy of my Medical Power of Attorney on file."

The orthopedic surgeon was there when the nurse made her announcement and the Scottish Warrior Princess fully took over my persona. The princess noticed a genuinely perplexed expression on the surgeon's face. I knew the woman was only doing her job. Very precisely, and to excess, in my view. *Can we say anal three times in a row?*

The Warrior Princess took a deep breath. Her voice was low and guttural; smoke was coming out of her ears.

"My mother and I have been using this hospital since 2004. She had two surgical procedures three years ago; she has been in the hospital three whole days at this point.

"Now is NOT the moment to inquire about Power of Attorney," the Warrior Princess said on my behalf. Her language was precise; her tone had a do-not-mess-with-me quality to it.

The surgeon disappeared. *Couldn't blame him for that*, and the Warrior Princess continued to roll. The nurse pressed the issue by calling her supervisor. By this time, the Princess was primal. I don't remember clearly the words that were exchanged or precisely how it came about. But, my mother went to surgery. I did NOT go home to produce a Medical Power of Attorney sheet of paper. I think I might have been too angry even to say vile, despicable words. At least, I don't remember saying them. I don't think I yelled. However, I did remember that someone told me once that I was scarier when I said things quietly, but firmly.

As I reported the story by email to family and friends, Cousin Pamela Garrett noted that circumstances with Miss Dixie weren't bad enough. "They needed to add some torture" to the scenario. *Indeed.*

During and after surgery, I stretched out on the sofa in the hospital room, and the sound of her breathing was a comfort. It seemed like home. It was what I listened for in the middle of the night. In the morning, I went home for a shower and to respond to messages, returning to find her awake and ready to eat. She ate the pureed diet heartily. And, she perked up.

"Barbara, let's get out of here," she said at one point.

She hadn't called me Barbara in two years, and I had to smile at her amazing ability to bounce back. After conferring with hospital staff, I dashed out to make arrangements to bring her home the next day. The prospect of full-time hospice nursing care for the first twenty-four hours lowered my anxiety level.

Another one of my pet peeves about Medicare equipment surfaced again. I had been trying to get a fully electric bed for the last few months. There were functions of the bed that didn't work properly. Since I now owned the bed, I was told by the vendor that fixing MY semi-electric bed would cost roughly $300 and no, I could not get a fully electric one through Medicare. It was irrelevant that cranking the bed up and down was killing my back. Actually, it made me laugh. Since I was now on Medicare, good old Medicare was going to pay for my bad back after the fact anyway. Delightfully bureaucratic irony there. Prevent it or fix it later? Take your pick.

Under hospice care, Miss Dixie was eligible for a fully electric hospital bed. Everything had to be done quickly. I was trading off the old bed for which Medicare had paid an outrageous amount of money through its leasing practices and which I now owned. Did the vendor buy the bed from me? No, of course not. So, the medical equipment provider got back the bed that I technically owned without a dime coming to me. Now, this piece of junk would be recycled to another unsuspecting Medicare recipient and Medicare would pay for a lease that would exceed the market price by at least three times its value. What a silly game. And the vendor got my good mattress, too, since I didn't have a place to store it. There may be cost efficiencies for Medicare to do business this way, but those efficiencies were hard for me to comprehend. And the medical equipment provider was added to my list of old people con games. Authorized theft.

Despite everyone's best efforts, Miss Dixie's departure was delayed. It was almost dark by the time she rolled into the house. Always before, her homecomings added joy to our journey. This time, however, I was sad beyond description. My optimism about her recovery from her fall and surgery was gone. I was at the edge of despair, but still trying to fool myself.

*

On Saturday morning, I fixed Miss Dixie's breakfast. While the hospice nursing aide fed her, I hurried out to get groceries. I had not been shopping in a week. By the time I returned, she had taken a downhill turn and my shopping trip was unnecessary. She was no longer eating and the end, though days away, was looming. She was dying. No more denial. Time for the advance person to start planning the next step. The funeral.

Active Dying

"Mother was moved from terminal to actively dying," I wrote. It was October 28, 2010, and five days since Miss Dixie had come home in hospice care. When I saw that gurney with my mother on it coming up the driveway, I was sick to my stomach.

"Vital signs won't be taken again to reduce agitation. I've been actively helping the hospice nurses care for her." My notes differ only slightly from the shift notes.

For a while, a machine to suction mucous was used to reduce coughing. Several days before, the hospice people had said I needed to hire someone to help with the machine. I said, "I'll learn how to do it." And, I did.

Today, the licensed practical nurse (LPN) reported her heart rate was over 100 and her blood pressure was low. The registered nurse (RN) who came this morning said Mother had anywhere from zero to seventy-two hours. Medications—morphine, lorazepam, and atropine, if needed— were placed under her tongue. A patch to reduce secretions was ordered; the suction machine would not be used any more. Too harsh.

The RN said it was clear she was trying to let go; she didn't want to be touched. I was surprised by that since she had allowed me to touch the center of her forehead—a calming place that I learned in yoga—in a soothing way. It had worked in the hospital and at home to reduce agitation.

*

At shift change in Arlington, Miss Dixie's nurse said she had bounced back a little. Here I was again at another end-of-life. I couldn't see the change that the nurse saw. With the new shift, I had to give medications since the nurse was not licensed to dispense them. Morphine at 5 p.m. and lorazepam at 7 p.m.

End-of-life care should be easier this time, I told myself. *You've seen sorrow before.* I went back to my desk to work on the slideshow for Mother's funeral service. I was typically in my zone, trying to get something to work out, when the nurse said, "Come." It didn't register with me at first. It was not time for medication, I said to myself.

Then, it hit me and I flew to the bedside. Her last breath was at 8:21 p.m. Her skin was soft and exquisite, like it belonged to a teenager. I sobbed and sobbed. Later, I wondered why. For ten years I expected this. No: truthfully, for ten years I worked to push it back, away. Of course, I knew I couldn't, but I still tried. *Nuts. Completely crazy.* Then, I called some friends. Tito, my good friend since high school and my pretend family member, came to be with me as the hospice nurse came to sign the papers, and we waited for the funeral home.

Two women came. The hospice social worker had told me not to watch my mother leave the house. Truthfully, I was relieved with her instruction. I had told her how sad I felt when my mother was brought into the house for what I knew was the last time. I was sick; the emotional pain was so strong.

Tito closed the door so I couldn't see. For me, it was also important that she be covered with blankets, not put in a black bag as my father was. Blankets seemed kinder, gentler. Yes, for me.

A Beautiful Little Church in Clover, West Virginia

Two weeks later, a handful of people gathered at the little church at Clover Cemetery in West Virginia. It was such a sweet-looking place. Of course, it was embellished a bit: a few of Miss Dixie's prettiest paintings and a poster-size photo I took earlier. A quilt, handmade by my grandmother, covered her casket. It had patches of red. The last of the greatest generation of Garretts was to be buried. Miss Dixie's two surviving brothers, each younger than she, had both died in a matter of months before. Loman died just twenty-one days earlier than Miss Dixie. With his death, I had felt an oppressive foreboding for my mother. *She would not want to be the last, to stay longer than her colorful, charming siblings.*

My extended family and friends rolled into action. Garrett Cousin Kate Burbank saved the beautiful hanging ferns from her summer porch and recommended a catering team for food after the service. Kincaid Cousin Bob Arnott from Denver was the tech guy setting up the slides for the lunch following the service. My friend from the Alzheimer's support group, Linda Willen, drove with me to Spencer and Clover with Mother's paintings. A long-ago friend, Ann Jeffries Johnson, drove in from upstate New York. Ann had come to our house to stay with us at the age of four or five while her mother was treated for cancer. Two Garrett cousins, Frances and Eddie, drove in from Detroit, and Pamela Garrett came for several days from Houston. I had never met Eddie, and the last time I saw Pamela was roughly fifty years earlier when she was three. Kincaid Cousin David Arnott, from eastern Ohio, told of the time that my mother and dad came to him after his mother's death to invite him to live with us so that he could go to college and work if he needed to. I didn't exactly remember it. But when he said it, it seemed familiar. Grant and Dolores Colthrop, friends for more than fifty years, came from Michigan to sing and officiate at Mother's service.

"The souls of the departed were calling her to join them," Cousin Candace Westfall had said.

A small, but special, gathering. Each person brought a piece and a story of a life lived fully with goodness, passion, and entertaining foibles.

The foods, I remembered particularly, were the regional tastes of my childhood. Potato salad with sweet pickle, West Virginia green beans seasoned with bacon. Turkey and ham. It poured rain and we didn't go to the graveside. I was relieved. There was something about placing her in the ground that I dreaded to the point of physical illness. When my father died, I worried that he was cold despite the oppressive August heat. I didn't want to leave him there. But he had picked the place he wanted to be, he wanted the three of US to be, years before.

There was one last thing from my mother, who always liked to run the show. I couldn't believe it. Confusion delayed the start of the service. The casket rolled into the church behind the arriving guests. No, that wasn't the plan. She had played me *one* last time. I had to smile. My mother was LATE again. After years of my forced punctuality, she showed me.

Even then, I was thinking of the advice of the hospice social worker. "You need to help her let go," she told me. "Tell her you need her help. You need her to help you write the BOOK."

I closed her eulogy that day with, "Godspeed, Mother dear. Godspeed." Now the story is also told, almost.

ONE YEAR LATER

I've been sad and physically ill this week. Maybe my illness was related to a new medication. I immediately went back to the old one, and I'll try the new one again in a couple of weeks. Originally, I had scheduled a stress test for today, but re-scheduled it after I got sick.

I have been sadly aware of how alone in the world I am without Mother and Dad. I signed on to a new online dating thing a couple of weeks ago. There's one man I would like to talk with again and another who quickly became a tedious, boring presence. There was a dazzling Italian painter online, but he never seems to check his email. This guy appeared to be too good to be true. *He was.*

This morning I got up with a burst of energy, washed my bed linens, ran the vacuum, and got rid of a couple more boxes.

I'm still unpacking boxes from my move. I got my house ready to sell in the spring, sold it in five days, bought a two-bedroom condo, gutted a perfectly useable though ugly kitchen, gutted two depressing bathrooms, and lived in a motel that smelled damp and moldy for three months, moving to a different room every twenty-eight days. I gained ten pounds eating junk from the machines, trying to soothe my sadness with food.

I have dreaded this anniversary because there is such hole in my life. My life's purpose is gone, though I have managed to numb myself by staying busy and have even tried to create a new purpose—building awareness about the family caregiving experience. I have a long presentation in Williamsburg next week.

The twice-a-month meetings of my Alzheimer's caregiver's support group are still on my calendar. Sometimes there is an opportunity to share some insight from my experience, but more importantly, I like to believe that the notion of "a life after caregiving" gives some hope to those still on the journey. Besides, giving back is a strong tradition with this particular group.

I just learned that my Michigan storefront property is vacant again. I was counting on that income. It looks like I need to continue to be very careful about expenses.

I just checked today's horoscope. I kid you not. This is what it said:

"Being forgetful can sometimes be a blessing—remember that the next time you're in a rush and you can't find your house keys or sunglasses. The same brain that makes you forget where you put something also lets you forget about hurtful episodes from your life—eventually. The pain or sorrow you've felt recently is fading slowly, but it's fading surely. Have faith that the worst is behind you, because it is. Keep moving forward, and leave the past behind."

MOUNTAINEERS, TIGERS, AND DREAMS

From time to time, I find strength and comfort in passages from *The Invitation* by Oriah Mountain Dreamer. I see it as the song of caregivers.

> *... I want to know*
> *if you can sit with pain*
> *mine or your own*
> *without moving to hide it*
> *or fade it*
> *or fix it.*

> *... I want to know if you can get up*
> *after the night of grief and despair*
> *weary and bruised to the bone*
> *and do what needs to be done...*

> *... I want to know*
> *if you can be alone*
> *with yourself*
> *and if you truly like*
> *the company you keep*
> *in the empty moments.*[24]

Strength and brutal honesty about who you are and what you can do. That's what it takes to give care.

---

24. Oriah Mountain Dreamer, "The Invitation," in *The Invitation* (San Francisco: HarperONE, 1999). All rights reserved. Presented with permission of the author. www. oriah.org.

December 1, 2013. I turned right just before the pretty, white country church, the church that held my mother's funeral. It was Sunday and there were a few cars, a little too early for the service. The road, really just a one-way path, was unpaved and bumpy, curving behind the church. The sky was dreary and the ground and trees showed the colors of winter. The hill was dotted with tombstones, some Garretts and Kincaids among them. The drop on the right side of the one-lane path seemed treacherous to these out-of-town eyes. Old Clover Cemetery was on the higher side of the hill, and a newer section sloped steeply down. Recent rains left deep puddles in the path, wanting gravel.

Sometimes Mother and Dad visit me in dreams. So far, they are always young, in their thirties and forties. I wonder why. Sometimes in my dream I'm in a terrible hurry to get someplace so that I can care for them, even though they're still young. I'm relieved when I wake that I haven't missed anything important. Very relieved.

I sold our/my two-generation house quickly because I needed to unload the mortgage and downsize myself. I now remember looking out Miss Dixie's hospital window, after her last surgery, at the tall buildings on a high piece of ground off in the distance, a few miles from the hospital. I had no idea at the time, but that's where I live now. Wonderfully, it took lots of focus to get through renovations in my new downsized apartment home. There were emotional crashes along the way. After my second contractor blew me off, I spent a day in bed curled into a fetal position. Healing. Resting until I could gather the strength to move ahead. Eventually, things got done—grief counseling helped. Before a year was up, I had a place to live that worked for me.

In the morning when I wake up, the first thing that I see is a painting by my mother. The snow is tinged with blue. The trees are white birch alongside a barn and windmill. Here and there are some leftover bright fall leaves in yellow with a touch of red. The painting is very Dixie. It's a winter scene but her colors are warm and vibrant, not the chill that comes from some frosty winter scenes. And, my father's handsome 1950s movie star photo looks down on me from the guest room. Both parents are present in that room. In my head, it's like they are still in Michigan. The urge to call them, to talk to them is ever present. The pain and sorrow happens when I admit that I can't. Away, but not forgotten.

Once, while talking to myself, I noted that Dixie and Hiram had not seen my new apartment and I needed to fix that oversight. That malfunction startled me, but I could also laugh at it.

This year I sold the Michigan storefront and little rental house. For me, this was much harder than selling the house Mother and Dad lived in for forty years or the house in Arlington that I had owned for thirty years. My attachment no longer made sense from a business perspective. I was too far away to manage it properly. But the emotional attachment was still there. I used to dream about spending time in the little house in the summers and revisiting my past. That was the place where I used to throw a purple comforter on my back and become the Queen of England. Where I remembered delirium when I had whooping cough. Where my dad mistakenly knocked a hole in the wall during heavy rains and made us temporarily homeless when the place flooded. And, where Mother put freshly picked zinnias on our summer kitchen table. It was the homely basement shelter of my childhood, not the big house my mother and dad loved.

At the cemetery, it took me two years to get it together enough to visit the graves. The sorrow had always felt too fresh. There was rawness that I was now alone. An only. A sole survivor. The thing I had dreaded most since childhood. The end of this family line. No need to worry about passing family photos and mementos on to my next generation. The end was here.

So, I began making active claims to other family lines: Lucille Garrett Johnson, the first Alzheimer's family caregiver that I ever knew. She was my caregiving model. My mother's sister and best friend. Her daughters, Kate and Candace, and their families, children and grandchildren were my new place of family belonging. My need for the bond as a part of my wholeness was still alive. What was it about my desire to physically be in West Virginia? I'm still searching. My mother and father both loved West Virginia in the way that I loved and appreciated Michigan. Although I missed the family connections of the state, I used to tell my mother and dad how grateful I was that they moved me to Michigan. How can you both love a place and be glad not to be there? I don't know, but I was and am.

Now, I love to go back to West Virginia for Thanksgiving. Whether it's twenty-three or twenty-six family members for dinner, I feel my heritage in that dining room. Three generations of strong capable women are seated in Candace's welcoming farmhouse. There are some terrific fellows around the tables, too. But the women blow your socks off.

Engaged, fierce mothers. Like my mother, a Mountaineer Tiger Woman. There's a doctor, speech therapist, former teacher, community activist, and healthcare activist.

In the youngest generation, Lucille, a teenager, already bears some characteristics of her great-grandmother. She's edging toward six feet tall, just like her namesake. Lucille, her older sisters, and cousins are already leaders. Rebekah, a skilled gymnast, will be fifteen when the Olympics roll around, and we might see her there. Lucille always gets a deer in hunting season, and sometimes she's the only one who does. This year Sarah, a fifth grader, got two deer, the legal limit. Of course, the boys got deer, too. There was talk of switching to bow and arrow next year.

We have buried the last of the Greatest Generation, but fear not. There are new generations to come.

EPILOGUE

Aging Child of Alzheimer's

As an aging child of Alzheimer's, I care deeply about biomedical research. I want good research and fast action. Preferably in the next ten years. Since I have also been a fundraiser and strategic planning consultant for nonprofit organizations, I have strongly held views about what will be needed to achieve Alzheimer's research breakthroughs.

Energy must come from the private, probably nonprofit sector. Government is too broken to lead, though government must be a partner.

Small, sharply focused nonprofits will provide the leadership. Yes, size does matter. Smaller is better. Large healthcare nonprofits tend to have mission creep, believing they must do everything for everyone. Focus, focus, focus.

Agility to move quickly in a changing environment will be essential. As of 2014, the failure rate of new Alzheimer's medication clinical trials suggests a crisis. One notable source puts it at more than ninety percent.

As a donor/investor in the most promising research approach, I check a nonprofit organization's Internal Revenue Service 990 before I invest. If I have trouble finding a 990, I don't invest. If I have trouble locating individual management salaries, I don't invest. If I find a nonprofit CEO with compensation in excess of a million dollars, I don't invest. When a cure is found, I may reconsider my personal compensation rule. But now? NO!

Yes, my rules are biased. There is no room for self-satisfaction and self-congratulation. I want systematic progress. I want a better understanding of the dynamics of the disease, better medications, and a cure. My rules are my rules. Follow them, or not. People, it's long past the time to kick it into gear. Everyone over the age of fifty is looking down the gun barrel of this disease, and the gun is loaded. That includes me.

"I know. But I do not approve. And I am not resigned."[25]

25. Edna St. Vincent Millay, "Dirge Without Music" in *Collected Poems*, edited by Norma Millay (Harper & Row, 1956).

APPENDICES

Notes for Family Caregivers

The Diagnosis and Later

The Alzheimer's Association uses a concise definition of the disease: Alzheimer's is a type of dementia that causes problems with memory, thinking, and behavior. Symptoms usually develop slowly and get worse over time, becoming severe enough to interfere with daily tasks.[26]

First, find a neurologist experienced in memory disorder diagnosis and treatment. Not all are.

Diagnostic Tests

There is no single widely used, absolute Alzheimer's test. Other possible causes of symptoms are eliminated.

Medications

Four medications, approved by the US Food and Drug Administration, treat Alzheimer's currently. Donepezil (Aricept®), rivastigmine (Exelon®), or galantamine (Razadyne®) are used to treat mild to moderate Alzheimer›s (donepezil can be used for severe Alzheimer›s as well). Memantine (Namenda®) is used to treat moderate to severe Alzheimer's.[27]

---

26. "What is Alzheimer's?" Alzheimer's Association, accessed April 2015, http://www.alz.org/alzheimers_disease_what_is_alzheimers.asp.

27. "About Alzheimer's Disease: Treatment," National Institute on Aging, accessed December 2014, http://www.nia.nih.gov/alzheimers/topics/treatment#drugs.

Antidepressants and anticonvulsants may also be prescribed to treat behavioral symptoms.[28]

Antidepressants include:

- Celexa® (Sa-LEKS-a), brand name; citalopram (SYE-tal-oh-pram), generic name

- Remeron® (REM-er-on), brand name; mirtazepine (MUR-taz-a-peen), generic name

- Zoloft® (ZO-loft), brand name; sertraline (SUR-truh-leen), generic name

Anticonvulsants, sometimes used to treat severe aggression, include:

- Depakote® (DEP-uh-cote), brand name; sodium valproate (so-DEE-um VAL-pro-ate), generic name

- Tegretol® (TEG-ruh-tall), brand name; carbamazepine (KAR-ba-maz-ee-peen), generic name

- Trileptal® (tri-LEP-tall), brand name; oxcarbazepine (oks-kar-BAZ-eh-peen), generic name

For guidance on sleeping aids and antipsychotic medications, please see the National Institute on Aging website for publications on Alzheimer's medications.

Preventative Medications

Currently none, though media reports periodically hype new possibilities.

Preventive Practices

Daily physical exercise and a healthy diet are urged, but there are numerous examples where healthy lifestyle practices have not prevented the onset of Alzheimer's.

---

28. "Caring for a Person with Alzheimer's Disease: Your Easy-to-Use Guide from the National National Institute on Aging," National Institute on Aging, accessed December 2014, http://www.nia.nih.gov/alzheimers/publication/medical-side-ad/medicines-treat-ad-symptoms-and-behaviors#behavior.

Activities of Daily Living

- Bathing

- Dressing

- Toileting

- Walking and other mobility issues, e.g. transfer movements from bed to chair.

- Eating

These activities are often the measurements of care that are referred to by healthcare professionals in evaluating where a patient is on the Alzheimer's continuum.

Services that help patients stay at home longer

Adult Day Care

Often initiated as respite care for family caregivers, adult day care has many additional benefits—socialization, friendships, and stimulating activities that engage and reward success to enrich the human existence of the Alzheimer's patient. But, it won't work for all patients.

Caregiving Support Groups

Support groups can help as informal advisors for sharing information on quality services and individuals in your area. The power of being heard cannot be understated as an empowerment tool. However, human nature and a tendency to vent in excess can undermine a group's usefulness. Trust your intuitive judgment to find the right group for you.

Products that Helped

I was an Internet shopper. I even got a new mattress for the Medicare-issued bed delivered to the house from the Internet. Medicare did not pay for it, of course. (The vendor should have been ashamed to issue the old mattress, as mentioned.)

- *Keyed dead bolt locks for exterior doors*

- *Washable plastic and cotton bed and chair liners*
- *Nightgowns* that snap at the top and are open down the back
- *Shirts* that open down the back
- *Large washable bibs* with Velcro at the neckline, long enough to also protect the lap
- *Adult diape*rs in different sizes—I ordered diapers from the Internet, also, largely because I had an aversion to driving all over town checking the big box stores for sizes and styles.
- *Travel wheelchairs*—I found one with the brakes on the handles. It helped my back.
- *Gait belt*—I learned about this great piece of equipment in a class. It's a fleece-lined belt that has several different strategically placed handgrips. This particular one is called the Assure Safety Transfer Belt, offered on the Internet by North Coast Medical. Like everything else in Alzheimer's family care, it worked very well until it didn't.
- *Shower chair with back support*—This was recommended by an occupational therapist and it was a terrific concept. It was ordered from the Internet.

Products We Tried but Didn't Work for Us

- Safe return bracelet
- Bed alarm
- Handle for car door

Just because they didn't work for us doesn't mean they might not work for you. So much of Alzheimer's care is still trial and error.

Family Caregiving Survival Lessons

Here are some basic survival tactics. Most come from my experience and that of my Alzheimer's Support Group.

- **If you've seen one case of Alzheimer's, you've seen ONE case!**

- **Take care of your own physical and mental health, first.** You can't afford to fall apart.

- **Get your legal ducks in a row.** We were lucky. We had done all of this before Alzheimer's kicked in noticeably. That's wills, power of attorney, and in some places an additional medical power of attorney. A lawyer who specializes in elder care law is an asset. Some may wish to specify in advance what care should take place near the end of life. Obviously, these decisions need to be made early when cognitive skills are still functioning. You may need a separate IRS power of attorney for tax filing while the patient can still write his/her name.

- **Do the research and take charge.** Learn about the disease. The medications. And, the right questions to ask of healthcare providers. Websites of the National Institute of Health and its associated organizations provide wonderful reliable information. The Alzheimer's Association and AARP (for caregiving) have great information, too. But, don't forget—stupid thrives on the web. Remember to rely on trusted websites.

- **Start the day taking care of yourself**. Get up early so you have some time for yourself. For me, it was riding on my recumbent bike. Why start the day? That's the only way it worked for me. Waiting until evening meant I was too tired and I never got to it.

- **Trial and error** is still the best operational tactic from medications to services.

- **Don't fight**. Even the most docile Alzheimer's patients will have confrontational moments. Leave the room to change the energy in it before you lose your temper. I failed at this several times before I learned to do it no matter what.

- **Don't explain too much**. Not always, but as the patient advances into the depths of Alzheimer's—what's the point of trying to explain something? Cognitive skills are gone. So, when the hospital tech tells the patient to relax, recognize that it's the tech's problem, not the patient's. If you are brave, try to initiate a teachable moment for the tech. Otherwise, breathe deeply for **your** blood pressure.

- **Don't get annoyed at the patient's behavior**. It's the disease, not the patient jerking you around. This sounds simple and obvious, but especially in the early years my mother drove me nuts with repetitive questions on the phone. Since I was hundreds of miles away in my happy little cocoon, it took me a long time to figure out it was Alzheimer's. Now, I know that it was the disease, not my mother trying to drive me nuts. Also, think of the disease as lying, not the patient.

- **Keep a journal and write emails and letters**. I have often kept a journal during difficult times. I was always amazed at how much I forgot when I went back to read it, but that's the point. Get it out. Put it on paper. Move on. Sometimes I wrote letters just for the pure entertainment value for me. Other times, I meant what I said. You know who you are out there. And sometimes I actually sent letters that I should not have sent.

- **Minor medical issues**, yours and the patient's, can compound and escalate quickly and exponentially in Alzheimer's care.

- **Find medical people you like and trust**. Stupid still happens, but it is less annoying and easier to forgive if you like the folks you are dealing with.

- **Fire the medical folks who refuse to hear what you are saying**. Very few medical professionals have done hands-on caregiving. So, don't expect that his or her medical training means he or she understands what you are dealing with or going through. Think of them as technical advisors and dispensers of prescriptions, keeping in mind that you may need to ask about specific medications for aggression, anxiety, and depression, in addition to the basic Alzheimer's medications. And if they don't think of it, it's up to you to ask.

- **Learn to pretend**. Some folks get all uptight about entering the unreality of the Alzheimer's patient's world. I came to think of it as a play opportunity. Of course, it's also known as lying. Get over your reticence. I was never all that impressed with reality anyway. So, play with it. Add some joy to the patient's life and yours.

- **Pick your battles**. Since you already know not to argue with the patient – sometimes the patient will resist necessary encounters with healthcare providers, for example. Is the appointment absolutely necessary? Maybe, maybe not.

- **Let it slide?** Some previously important health tasks and protocols may not be necessary. A colonoscopy? Really? Treatment decisions for potentially terminal diseases, such as cancer, are extremely complicated. Misery versus quality of life—very difficult balance.

- **Trust your intuitive judgment**. This applies to healthcare providers and solutions for caregiving dilemmas.

- **Self-correction** will be your most useful tool. You can't change the patient, but you can change YOURSELF and the way you react and respond.

- **Focus on today and now.** Life will be easier if you do.

- **Learn to forgive yourself**. It's likely that there will be several occasions when you will say to yourself: "Why didn't I see that before?" So, big deal. You're human and mistakes happen. Maybe you were tired.

- **Grief** over a long period of time is a significant element of family caregiving. There may be grief for the person who was, as well as grief for the impact of caregiving on your life. It seems obvious, but, of course, it can mess with your psyche in unexpected ways.

- **Show up**. As one of our support group leaders said, "Sometimes showing up is all you can do." With Alzheimer's, showing up can take guts. The grief counselors call it "bearing witness." It is important to surround the dying with love and support if possible. Isn't that what we all would hope to have? Showing up is guts and class all rolled into one for Alzheimer's family members. Remember, this thing may run in the family.

Resources for Alzheimer's Family Caregivers

Government Websites

- National Institute on Aging. http://www.nia.nih.gov/Alzheimers/. Authoritative definitions and up-to-date information on the disease and research progress on this disease for which there is no cure.

- The Alzheimer's Disease Education and Referral (ADEAR) Website. http://www.nia.nih.gov/Alzheimers/AlzheimersInformation/AboutUs.htm. Good information, and you can sign up to get press release on breaking news associated with Alzheimer's.

Organization Websites

- Alzheimer's Association. http://www.alz.org Excellent information on the disease, caregiving, and especially the stages of Alzheimer's (http://www.alz.org/alzheimers_disease_stages_of_alzheimers.asp). Local chapters may sponsor caregiving support groups, which can be very helpful and supportive.

- AARP Caregiving Resources Center. http://www.aarp.org/relationships/caregiving/ Toolkits and publications on a range of issues including legal and financial issues. Compassion and Choices. https://www.compassionandchoices.org/what-we-do/advance-directive/ Can help with language in advance directives for end-of-life care for dementia patients.

- National Alliance for Caregiving. http://www.caregiving.org/ Some caregiving information, but general research information on the impact of family caregiving on individuals, corporations, etc. General caregiving, not just Alzheimer's.

- Cure Alzheimer's Fund. http://curealz.org/ A relatively new organization focused on supporting scientific research that promises to lead to a cure. Detailed reports on studies that are readable for non-scientists.

- Family Caregiver Alliance. http://www.caregiver.org/caregiver/jsp/home.jsp Originally a community-based organization that has expanded its reach nationally. Provides high-quality information for caregivers of many diseases in addition to Alzheimer's.

- Fisher Center for Alzheimer's Research. http://www.alzinfo.org. Contains articles that are peer reviewed by Alzheimer's researchers.

Books/Publications

How-To-Care

- *The 36-Hour Day: A Family Guide of Caring for Persons* by Nancy Mace and Peter Y. Rabins. A must-have primer for family caregiving.

- *Learning to Speak Alzheimer's* by Joanne Koenig Coste. Became my favorite Alzheimer's book because it emphasized working with where the patient is.

- *Alzheimer's Early Stages: First Steps for Family, Friends and Caregivers* by Daniel Kuhn with a foreword by David A. Bennett, MD.

- *Coach Broyles' Playbook for Alzheimer's Caregivers* by Frank Broyles. Very readable, full of good advice, and available as a free download or as a printed book for a modest cost. Also can be found on the Alzheimer's Association Website.

- *Red Cross Family Caregiving Reference Guide*. Available as a download or printed book. Shows how to safely move a patient, etc.

Memoirs

- *Losing My Mind* by Thomas DeBaggio. A sad, moving story by an herb grower, former journalist as he begins his journey into early onset Alzheimer's.

- *Don't Eat the Elephants* by Patricia H. Miller. Love story and how-to book all in one.

- *Jan's Story* by Barry Petersen. A stunning portrait of a marriage and life devastated by early onset Alzheimer's.

- *Slow Dancing with a Stranger* by Meryl Comer. A powerful story of early onset Alzheimer's failed diagnosis and twenty years of caregiving.

Other Web Sources

- Caring.com. http://www.caring.com/ Founded in 2007, provides expert advice on range of issues directly related to Alzheimer's family care. Also has steps and stages advice. Join for regular email messages.

- A Place for Mom.com. http://www.aplaceformom.com/ A referral service that includes care homes that often work for patients in need of a non-institutional environment. Also has email messages on caregiving.

- Alzheimer's Reading Room.com. http://www.alzheimersreadingroom.com/ Website and blog, succinct source of useful caregiving advice and health information for the Alzheimer's community. The founder cared for his mother and started writing about what he learned. Currently my favorite source of credible experience...

- A compelling and beautifully written blog by David Hilfiker, a Washington, DC, resident who was diagnosed with Alzheimer's in 2012. For best results in a Google search, paste the title into your browser, "Watching the Lights Go Out: A Memoir from inside Alzheimer's Disease."

*

Compiled and recommended by Barbara K Kincaid, an Alzheimer's family caregiver in Northern Virginia for ten years. Prepared for

Genesis Rehab Services 11/4/2011. *Updated annually for use by Alzheimer's Support Group, Arlington, VA with additions by support group members.*

ACKNOWLEDGMENTS

So many have helped along the way. Author D. W. Buffa, also a long-time friend from my days in politics, was my developmental editor. He didn't plan to do it, but that's what he did. His specific advice on my book and his knowledge of book publishing helped significantly. His guidance was instrumental in getting my memoir "over the wall," as we used to say in politics. Nothing counts if it doesn't get over the wall. He also had met both of my parents, resulting in a good sense of the subject matter.

Fortuitously, I joined a memoir writers group in April 2012. The group was led by Bonnie Demars. She moved to Boston and Marcia Molina (Mayu) Lehmann took the lead. Both were superb leaders and good friends whose thoughtful commentary gave comfort and support throughout the process. The memoir group spanned the decades in terms of ages, and their feedback helped provide clarity through multi-generational eyes and ears. Special thanks to Margaret Anthony, Janet Barber, Ann H. Tran Cruz, and Moira McGuinness for cheering me on literally for years.

And, the cousins. So many times I would have been a lost and drifting soul without my Kincaid and Garrett cousins. These connections began when I was just beginning to walk. They were playmates at family reunions and my first friends. As lives got busy, contact diminished, but was easily restored as we got older and were able to make more time. Special thanks to Bob and Dolores Arnott, Kate and Bill Burbank, Pam Garrett and Ernie Simien, and Candace and Jim Westfall.

Different drafts of the book were "workshopped" in classes sponsored by Politics & Prose Bookstore in Washington, DC, and The Writers' Center in Bethesda, MD. Thanks to the Politics memoir manuscript class, which reviewed a first draft and provided ideas that became important parts to the book in later drafts. Special thanks also to author and Writers' Center instructor Maxine Clair for feedback on the pieces, which unraveled the emotion and helped with clarity.

Teacher Johanna Scharmen, my 11th grade English teacher, is probably the one to whom I owe the most. She tagged me with, "I know. But I do not approve. And I am not resigned." The line is from Edna St Vincent Millay's "Dirge Without Music." She chose a line of poetry for everyone in our high school graduating class. Her choice for me turned out to be a remarkable character analysis, which I hated, of course, and spent pretty much every minute of my life living. Then, there was the late Harry B. Stapler, editor and publisher of the East Lansing Towne Courier in East Lansing, Michigan. As my boss, he was a great writing and editing instructor, perhaps the best I ever had. He also urged me to trust my "first instinct," as he called it. You get in trouble, he said, when you start over-thinking things. Still happens, I'm sorry to say.

Of course, I must mention the world's greatest family caregivers support group. There have been so many members that I dare not name them for missing one. Here are some facilitators/leaders to whom I am most grateful: William Kays, the late Alan Dirkson, John A. (Andy) Spanogle Jr., Linda Willen, Helen Horton, Kathy Ferger, and Liz Wheeler.

There were and are many other friends who made the journey possible. They are identified on the pages of the book as my thanks for their generosity and kindness.

REVIEW

COME LIVE WITH ME
A Memoir of Family, Alzheimer's, and Hope
Barbara K. Kincaid
September 30, 2015

In this luminous debut memoir, a woman struggles to care for her
Alzheimer's-stricken mother, experiencing exhaustion, heartache,
moments of joy, and a renewed connection to her loved ones.

Kincaid, an only child who never married, spent a decade caring
for her mother, Dixie Garrett Kincaid, after she began suffering
from dementia, eventually taking her into her own Arlington,
Virginia, home. As the disease progressed from forgetfulness to
eccentricity to a loss of reason, self-control, and language, the
author found herself becoming a parent to her mother, whom she
often characterizes as being as helpless and demanding as an infant,
yet big and mobile enough to cause chaos. Kincaid is unsparing
about the realities of Alzheimer's care, describing her mother's
hygiene problems and violent outbursts; her sometimes-charming,
sometimes-infuriating habit of hiding clothes and household
objects; and her recurrent medical emergencies, exacerbated by her
inability to explain what was wrong. The author also describes her
own sleep deprivation and her feelings of intense guilt when she
had to deposit her mother in respite care to let herself recuperate.
She cogently criticizes the nationwide Alzheimer's-care network for
its frequent lapses and callousness, castigates doctors for making
cavalier treatment decisions without considering her mother's
circumstances, and accuses a nursing facility of making false
medical claims to justify sending her mother back to the hospital.

The author's wrangles with HMO doctors to get treatment for her own serious ailments, including breast cancer, constitute an appalling health care horror story of its own. But there are also rewards here: her mother's once-difficult temperament improves as she experiences happiness, satisfaction, and episodes of clarity, and Kincaid's caregiving results in a deeper familial bond. The author sets the story of her care against description of her fraught relationship with her mother before her decline, and of the strong, inspirational women in her extended family. In vivid, graceful prose, she offers an honest account of the burdens of Alzheimer's patients without losing sight of their importance in the lives of those who care for them.

A cleareyed, moving portrait of Alzheimer's and the family ties that transcend it.

- Kirkus Review (starred review)

Made in the USA
Columbia, SC
21 November 2017